Fiberoptic Endoscopy in Anesthesia

FIBEROPTIC ENDOSCOPY IN ANESTHESIA

VIJAYALAKSHMI U. PATIL, M.D.
Instructor, Department of Anesthesiology
Upstate Medical Center
Syracuse, New York

LINDA C. STEHLING, M.D.
Professor of Anesthesiology and Pediatrics
Upstate Medical Center
Syracuse, New York

HOWARD L. ZAUDER, M.D., Ph.D.
Professor and Chairman, Department of Anesthesiology
Professor of Pharmacology
State University of New York
Upstate Medical Center
Syracuse, New York

Illustrations by VIJAYALAKSHMI U. PATIL, M.D.

YEAR BOOK MEDICAL PUBLISHERS, INC.
CHICAGO · LONDON

Copyright © 1983 by Year Book Medical Publishers, Inc. All rights reserved. No part of this publication may be reproduced, stored in a retrieval system, or transmitted, in any form or by any means, electronic, mechanical, photocopying, recording, or otherwise, without prior written permission from the publisher. Printed in the United States of America.

Library of Congress Cataloging in Publication Data
Patil, Vijayalakshmi U., 1940–
  Fiberoptic endoscopy in anesthesia.

  Includes index.
   1. Endoscope and endoscopy. 2. Trachea—Intubation.
3. Fiber optics. I. Stehling, Linda C., 1942–
II. Zauder, Howard L., 1923–   III. Title.
[DNLM: 1. Endoscopy. 2. Fiber optics. 3. Intubation, Intratracheal. WO 280 P298f]
RF476.P37 1983   616.2'307545   83-6752
ISBN 0-8151-6655-9

Contents

PREFACE vii

1 / HISTORICAL DEVELOPMENT AND OPTICAL PRINCIPLES 1
    History of Endotracheal Intubation 1
    Introduction of Fiberoptic Endoscopy 1
    Principles of the Fiberoptic Endoscope 2

2 / INSTRUMENTATION AND AUXILIARY EQUIPMENT 9
    Available Instrumentation 9
    Care of the Instrument 9
    Cleaning and Sterilization 10
    Ancillary Equipment 11
    Available Instrumentation 13
    Care of the Instrument 21
    Cleaning and Sterilization 26
    Ancillary Equipment 27

3 / PHARMACOLOGY OF ADJUVANT DRUGS 37
    Antisialagogues 37
    Vasoconstrictors 37
    General Anesthesia 37
    Local Anesthesia 39
    Intravenous Sedation 40

4 / ANATOMY FOR THE ENDOSCOPIST 43
    Sensory Innervation of the Airway 44
    Normal Airway Anatomy 46
    Airway of the Infant 69

5 / TECHNIQUES OF ENDOTRACHEAL INTUBATION 75
    Becoming Familiar with the Instrument 75
    The Technique 75
    Reasons for Failure 76
    Planning the Anesthetic 77
    Regional and Topical Anesthesia 77
    General Anesthesia 78
    Orotracheal vs. Nasotracheal Intubation 78
    Positioning the Patient 79
    Anticipating Difficulty with Intubation 79
    Unpredicted Difficulty with Endotracheal Intubation 80
    Complications and Precautions 80
    Gaining Facility with the Instrument 82
    Preparation of Equipment 83
    Placement of the Insertion Tube 87
    Reasons for Failure 97

    Nerve Block Techniques. 101
    Endoscopic Intubation Under General Anesthesia 103
    Endoscopic Intubation with Local Anesthesia 106
    Use of an Intubation Gauge 110
    Endoscopic Intubation in Children 113

6 / CLINICAL APPLICATIONS 115
    Evaluation of Airway Pathology 116
    Confirmation of Tube Placement 126
    Positioning Segmental Bronchial Blockers. 131
    Changing Endotracheal Tubes 135
    Performing Tracheobronchial Toilet 138
    Placing Nasogastric Tubes 140

Preface

FIBEROPTIC ENDOSCOPY has been available to the anesthesiologist for almost two decades yet it is not widely used. The inexperienced endoscopist usually blames the instrument for his or her own ineptness. Most anesthesiologists first attempt fiberoptic laryngoscopy after conventional laryngoscopy and endotracheal intubation have failed. Under such circumstances fiberoptic endoscopy is also usually unsuccessful and the instrument judged worthless and relegated to a back shelf.

There are numerous case reports extolling the merits of fiberoptic endoscopy in specific clinical situations. Manufacturers' brochures provide some information regarding care of the instruments. There is, however, no manual or text available to anesthesiologists interested in learning the technique. In response to this need, the authors have attempted to synthesize the information with which the clinician should be familiar before performing fiberoptic endoscopy.

The principles and components of fiberoptic endoscopes as well as step-by-step descriptions of their use are included. Success often is dependent upon seemingly minor details such as the manner in which the lens is defogged or lubricant is applied to the insertion tube. Ancillary equipment such as the Patil-Syracuse endoscopic mask and airway is detailed and its use illustrated. Although these mechanical aids are not essential to successful fiberoptic endoscopy, we have found that they facilitate the technique. Normal anatomy and several significant pathologic states are presented. Intubation models and cadavers were employed in situations where use of human subjects was not feasible. Most of the endoscopic photographs were taken through a pediatric fiberoptic bronchoscope and are easily distinguished from those in which an optical stylet was used. The latter, not a fiberoptic instrument, lacks the grid-like pattern produced by fiber bundles. To the novice, the grid or screen appearance is distracting; the experienced endoscopist hardly notices it.

Fiberoptic endoscopy appears deceptively simple when properly performed. However, facility with the instrument is gained only through practice. One must obtain initial experience by using the instrument in an intubation model, not patients. Next, the technique should be employed in patients with normal anatomy scheduled for elective operative procedures. Only after the endoscopist has become adept with the instrument should he or she perform fiberoptic endoscopy in patients with abnormal anatomy or in emergency situations.

The skilled endoscopist will find many uses for the technique, particularly in patients with craniofacial dysostoses, rheumatoid arthritis, morbid obesity, and deformities resulting from previous surgical procedures or burn scar contractures. Many patients, previously denied surgical procedures because endotracheal intubation was extremely difficult or impossible, can be intubated with the aid of fiberoptic endoscopy. Others can be spared the discomfort and trauma of awake intubation or the morbidity of tracheostomy. However, fiberoptic endoscopy is not a technique to be used only in patients in whom endotracheal intubation is difficult. Neither should the technique be considered a last resort. When difficulty with endotracheal intubation is anticipated, arrangements for fiberoptic laryngoscopy should be made in advance.

The techniques illustrated have proven useful in the authors' clinical practice. We do not imply that they represent the only approaches to given situations. The experienced endoscopist will find new applications and modifications of the technique.

We are grateful to American Optical and Olympus for photographs and use of instruments. The cooperation of our surgical colleagues is appreciated. Without the editorial and secretarial assistance of Ms. Diane Coe and Barbara Esposito this monograph would still be a disorganized mass of photographs and legends.

VIJAYALAKSHMI U. PATIL, M.D.
LINDA C. STEHLING, M.D.
HOWARD L. ZAUDER, M.D., Ph.D.

1 / Historical Development and Optical Principles

HISTORY OF ENDOTRACHEAL INTUBATION

WHILE INTUBATION of the trachea for purposes of resuscitation of experimental animals is three centuries older than anesthesia itself, endotracheal anesthesia, as we know it today, was conceived in Glasgow 100 years ago. Macewen[1] passed a rigid tube through the mouth guided by the sense of touch for an operative procedure on the base of the tongue. However, it was the classic work of O'Dwyer,[2] who intubated the trachea as a lifesaving maneuver in patients with diphtheria, that resulted in the evolution of contemporary endotracheal anesthesia. A number of physicians and physiologists in the United States and Europe experimented with rigid, semirigid, and soft tubes of both the cuffed and uncuffed variety that were introduced with one or more mechanical devices or were guided by the operator's tactile sense. While Kuhn[3] developed and applied most of the principles of endotracheal anesthesia in current use, it remained for others to refine and popularize the technique.

Indirect laryngoscopy was known and practiced in the first century A.D.; direct laryngoscopy appears to have originated in 1895.[4] The instrumentation and techniques of direct laryngoscopy so eloquently developed by Jackson were first applied to anesthesia by Elsberg.[5] Jackson[6] himself stressed the applicability of his developments to the needs of the anesthesiologist in 1913. That same year Janeway[7] described a laryngoscope with a curved blade attached to a handle containing a dry battery. Major advances in the techniques of endotracheal anesthesia occurred during WWI, when Robotham and Magill[8] made their monumental contributions. With the exception of a few modifications of endotracheal tube material, cuff design, and laryngoscope blades, no significant technical progress was made for half a century. The patient with a difficult airway who could not be intubated or safely managed with an anesthetic delivered by mask faced tracheostomy to establish and maintain the airway. A number of retrograde techniques, guides, and hooks were described as aids to intubation; all were at best traumatic and at worst uncertain.

INTRODUCTION OF FIBEROPTIC ENDOSCOPY

A new era dawned in 1963, when Murphy[9] utilized a fiberoptic choledochoscope to facilitate nasotracheal intubation. Four years later Taylor and Towey,[10] and Conyers et al.[11] reported the use of fiberoptic bronchoscopes to aid in the passage of nasotracheal tubes in patients with severe rheumatoid arthritis in whom conventional endotracheal intubation was impossible. The same year Stiles et al.[12] described the use of a flexible fiberoptic laryngoscope in a series of 100 patients, 20 of whom had severe limitation of movement of the cervical spine or temporomandibular joints. In 1973 Davis[13] reported the development, in conjunction with the American Optical Corporation, of a fiberoptic laryngoscope specifically designed to meet the needs of the anesthesiologist at a fraction of the cost of the fiberoptic bronchoscope. The following year Raj and associates[14] presented an analysis of the use of this new instrument in 50 patients. Their detailed description of the procedures applicable to both oral and nasal intubation resulted in widespread acceptance of this new technique. With the passage of time, the fiberoptic laryngoscope and bronchoscope have become indispensable parts of the anesthesiologist's armamentarium.

PRINCIPLES OF THE FIBEROPTIC ENDOSCOPE

When a glass rod is melted and rapidly stretched, the molten portion forms a long, fine, threadlike structure that loses most of the physical characteristics of glass. The fiber does, however, retain the ability to transmit light. It has long been recognized that if a beam of light enters one end-face of a glass rod, it is repeatedly reflected at the walls of the rod and emerges from the opposite

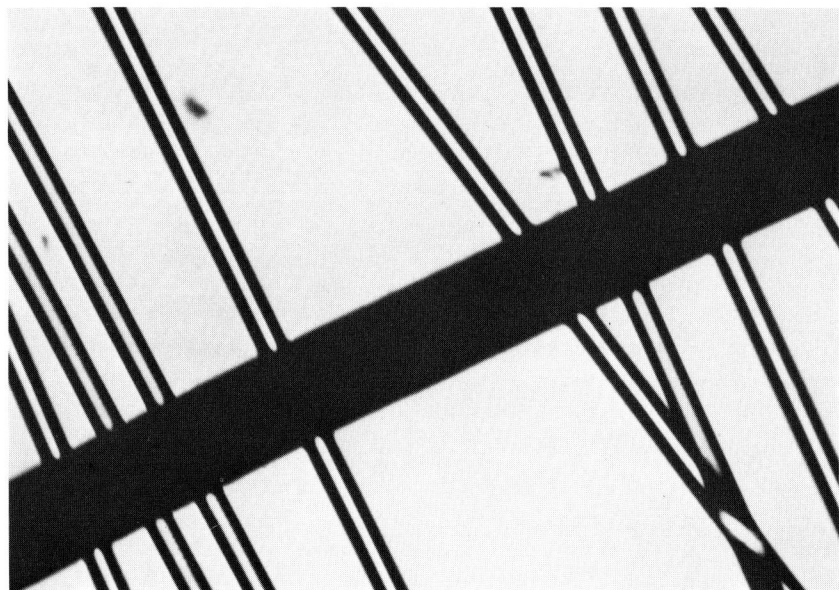

Fig 1–1.—Diameter of "clad" fibers relative to a human hair.

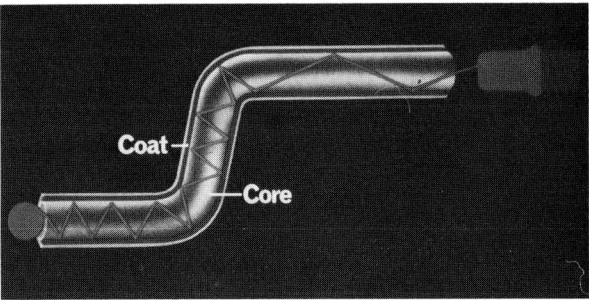

Fig 1–2.—Representation of the path taken by a beam of light entering and exiting a glass fiber.

end-face. Ideally, there would be total internal reflection with no light lost other than by absorption as the light waves travel between reflections through the glass. It is this trapping that results in transmission of the image. Fibers 5–25 μ in diameter not only transmit light and images but also are flexible. This flexibility, as well as the optical qualities of the fibers, was first described in the late 19th century. It was not until the 1920s and 1930s that the ability of flexible glass fibers to transmit light was put to a number of practical applications. In 1930 glass fibers were incorporated into a flexible gastroscope.

The fibers initially employed were not ideal in that significant light was lost from the surface of the fiber and thus was not totally internally reflected and transmitted from one end to the other. While the early instruments were

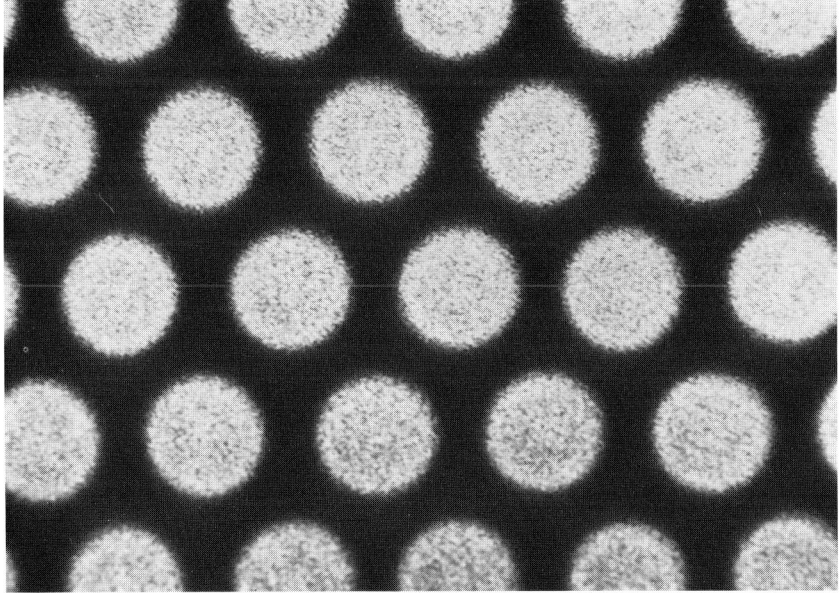

Fig 1–3.—Photomicrograph of fiber bundle.

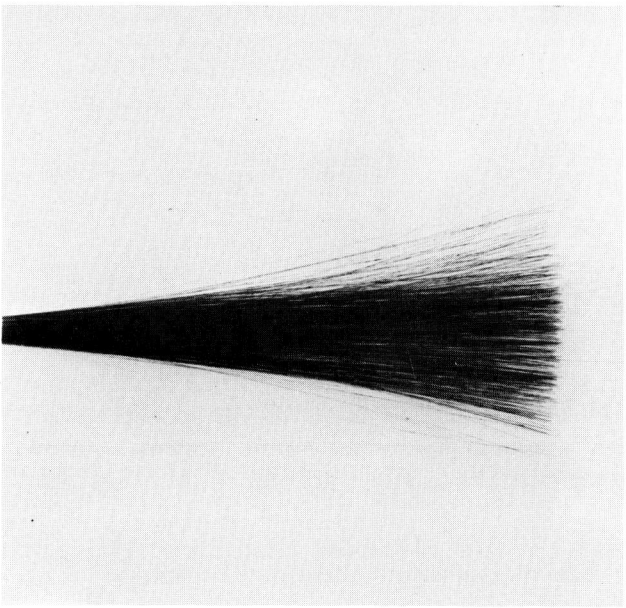

Fig 1-4.—Transverse section of unbound fiber bundle.

composed of bundles of fibers, optical insulation was not possible. Since 1950 it has been common to coat the glass fiber (core glass) with a thin exterior layer of glass (cladding glass) of a lower refractive index, thus effectively providing total optical insulation of each fiber in the bundle. Light entering the fiber at a specific angle of incidence at the end of the cut surface travels through the fiber, repeatedly striking and being reflected from the cladding glass at a similar angle of incidence until it emerges from the opposite cut surface. For fibers

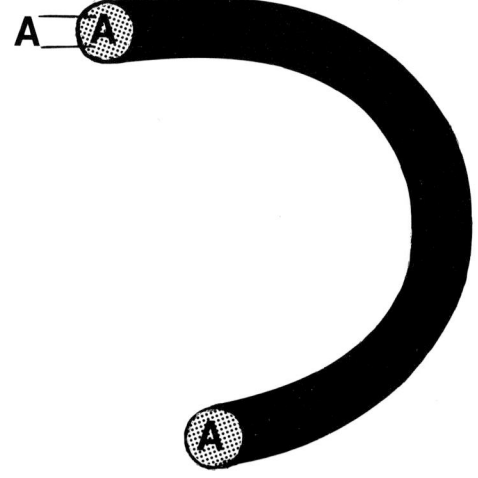

Fig 1-5.—Transmission of image by a coherent bundle.

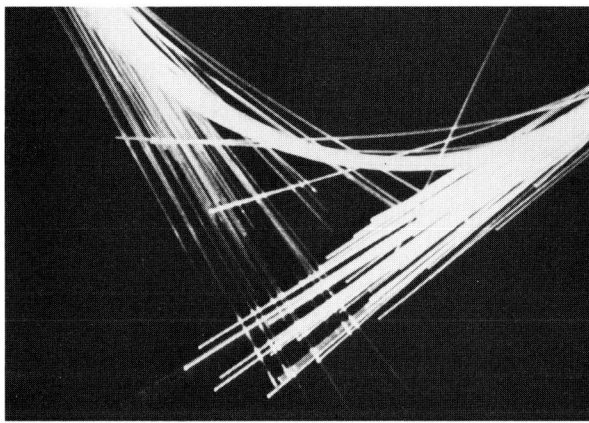

Fig 1–6.—Part of glass fiber bundle, magnified.

of the size commonly employed in an endoscope (Fig 1–1) the angle of incidence remains virtually constant when the fiber is bent within a limited radius (Fig 1–2). The incorporation of a number of such fibers into a bundle (Figs 1–3 and 1–4) forms the basis of the fiberscope.

There are two uses for bundles of fibers in the endoscope—the illumination of the surface to be examined and the transport of the image to the proximal portion of the instrument. Light from any of a number of sources is usually carried to the distal end of the instrument by bundles of fibers with diameters approximately 25 μ. No precise order or arrangement of fibers is necessary in the light-transmitting bundle (incoherent bundle). On the other hand, fibers in the image-transmitting bundle (coherent bundle) are somewhat smaller in diameter and must be arranged so that the ordering of fibers in the proximal end of the bundle coincides with the ordering of the same fibers at the distal end. Were this not the case, the image would be scrambled. If the bundle is coherent, each fiber will convey its image to the proximal end in strict accord with the light and shade viewed by the distal fibers (Fig 1–5). Each bundle consists

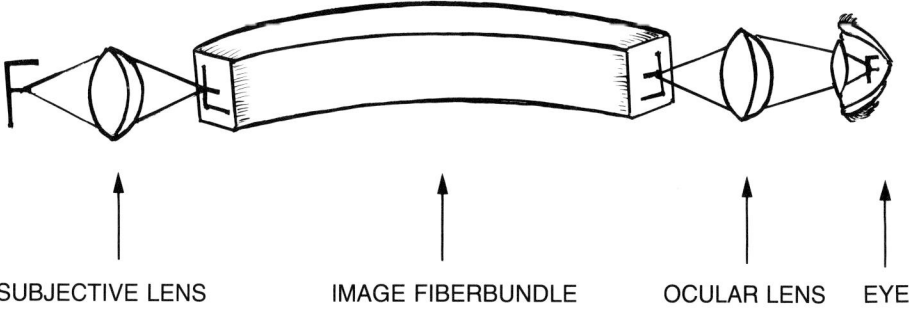

SUBJECTIVE LENS   IMAGE FIBERBUNDLE   OCULAR LENS   EYE

Fig 1–7.—The image, inverted by the distal lens, is restored to its proper orientation by the ocular lens.

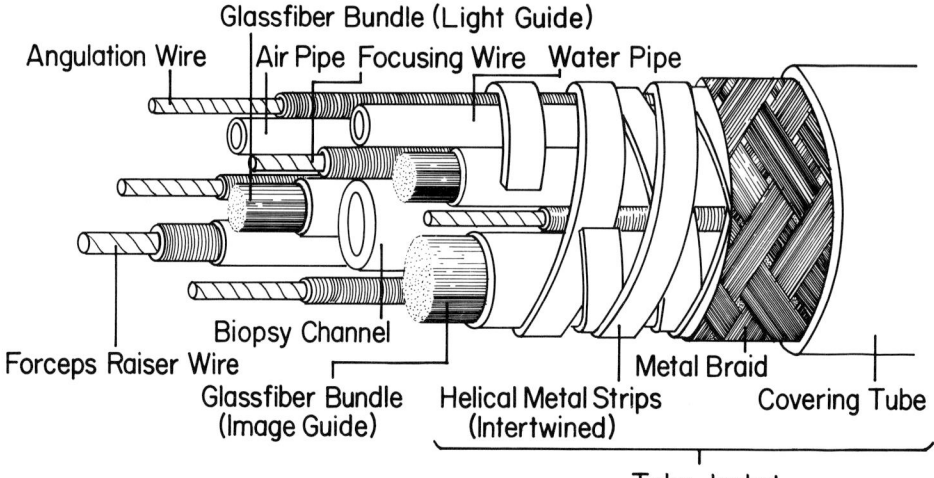

Fig 1–8.—Internal construction of insertion tube.

of between 10,000 and 15,000 fibers nearly identical in diameter and optical characteristics (Fig 1–6). Resolution is dependent entirely on the regularity, density, and compactness of the fibers at both ends. The smaller the fiber the better the resolution: should the fiber be too thin (less than 5 μ), strength and the ability to transmit light are lost. The pattern of fiber arrangement and the methodology employed to maintain the alignment of the fibers at the proximal and distal ends remain a trade secret.

When the cut ends of the bundles are polished, they are fitted with a series of lenses. The objective (distal lens) is used to focus the image on the distal end of the bundle. In accord with basic principles of optics, this inverts the image, which may be restored to proper orientation by rotating the bundle through 180 degrees or, more commonly, by fitting the proximal portion with a lens or eyepiece (Fig 1–7). This allows for magnification and the transmission of the image to a point where it may be conveniently viewed by the eye of the observer.

In its simplest configuration, the endoscope consists of two fiber bundles (light and image) and an angulation wire encased in metal braid that in turn is covered with a plastic sheath. The more complex instruments (Fig 1–8) contain, within the sheath, channels for suction or insufflation of oxygen or anesthetic mixtures, wires that permit focusing and forceps manipulation and, finally, a tube for the passage of diagnostic and therapeutic instruments.

REFERENCES

1. Macewen W.: Clinical observations on the introduction of tracheal tubes by the mouth instead of performing tracheotomy or laryngotomy. *Br. Med. J.* 2:122, 1880.
2. O'Dwyer J.: Fifty cases of croup in private practice treated by intubation of the

larynx with a description of the method and of the dangers incident thereto. *Med. Record* 52:557, 1887.
3. Kuhn F.: Die perorale intubation. *Zentralbl. Chir.* 28:1281, 1901.
4. Keys T.E.: *History of Surgical Anesthesia.* New York, Schumans, 1945, p. 68.
5. Elsberg C.A.: Intratracheal insufflation anesthesia; its value in thoracic and in general surgery. *N.Y. J. Med.* 12:524, 1912.
6. Jackson C.: The technique of insertion of intratracheal insufflation tubes. *Surg. Gynecol. Obstet.* 17:507, 1913.
7. Janeway H.H.: Intratracheal anesthesia from the standpoint of the nose, throat and oral surgeon with a description of a new instrument for catheterizing the trachea. *Laryngoscope* 23:1082, 1913.
8. Rowbotham E.S., Magill I.W.: Anaesthetics in the plastic surgery of the face and jaws. *Proc. R. Soc. Med. (Anaesth.)* 14:17, 1921.
9. Murphy P.: A fibre-optic endoscope used for nasal intubation. *Anaesthesia* 22:489, 1967.
10. Taylor P.A., Towey R.M.: The broncho-fiberscope as an aid to endotracheal intubation. *Br. J. Anaesth.* 44:611, 1972.
11. Conyers A.B., Wallace D.H., Mulder D.S.: Use of the fiberoptic bronchoscope for nasotracheal intubation: A case report. *Can. Anaesth. Soc. J.* 19:654, 1972.
12. Stiles C.M., Stiles Q.R., Denson J.S.: A flexible fiber-optic laryngoscope. *J.A.M.A.* 221:1246, 1972.
13. Davis N.J.: A new fiberoptic laryngoscope for nasal intubation. *Anesth. Analg.* 52:807, 1973.
14. Raj P.P., Forestner J., Watson T.D., et al.: Technics for fiberoptic laryngoscopy in anesthesia. *Anesth. Analg.* 53:708, 1974.

2 / Instrumentation and Auxiliary Equipment

FIBEROPTIC ENDOSCOPES vary in size, price, and available options. Some manufacturers will fabricate instruments to users' specifications. Prior to purchasing an endoscope, the anesthesiologist must consider the clinical situations in which the instrument will be employed, recognizing that it has uses other than endotracheal intubation. Ideally, the instrument is chosen on the basis of the options available (Table 2–1) and the type of patients with whom the anesthesiologist deals most frequently. For example, it makes little sense for the pediatric anesthesiologist to spend several thousand dollars on an instrument that can be used with nothing smaller than a 7-mm endotracheal tube.

AVAILABLE INSTRUMENTATION

Endoscopes and light sources range in price from a few hundred to several thousand dollars, depending on the quality of the optics and the options chosen. The basic components of the endoscope are the control section and insertion tube. Some are equipped with a suction channel that can also be used to insufflate oxygen and instill local anesthetic agents. Most have bending angles that range from 60 to 180 degrees in a vertical plane. The insertion tubes vary in length and diameter, determining the size of endotracheal tube that can be used. The image visualized depends in large part on the light source. Many operating rooms have fiberoptic light sources that can be used, obviating additional expenditure.

CARE OF THE INSTRUMENT

Fiberoptic endoscopes are delicate instruments and can easily be destroyed by careless handling. Damage to fiber bundles results in loss of the image or light in individual fibers, which cannot be repaired or replaced. Therefore, use of the instrument should be restricted to those who are familiar with its care.

It is best to store the endoscope in a padded case or well-padded drawer of an endoscopy cart. The insertion tube must never be tightly coiled or sharply bent. When applying an antifog agent to the lens, the insertion tube should be grasped distal to the angle bend and held firmly with the thumb and index finger. The end of the insertion tube must never be allowed to strike another object, because damage to the distal lens will result. Forcing the insertion tube into an endotracheal tube that is too small may damage the sheath or glass

TABLE 2–1.—FIBEROPTIC ENDOSCOPES

MANUFACTURER	OUTER DIAMETER (mm)	PERMISSIBLE ENDOTRACHEAL TUBE (I.D., mm)	BENDING ANGLE (degrees)	WORKING LENGTH (cm)	CHANNEL DIAMETER (mm)
Fiberoptic Stylet Laryngoscope					
American Optical SLS*†	5.6	6.5	Semiflexible except for distal 2.5 cm	28.5	None
Fiberoptic Rhinolaryngoscopes					
Olympus ENF-L	4.6	5.5	130 up / 90 down	41.0	None
Machida ENT-3L	3.3	4.0	100 up / 100 down	30.0	None
	4.0	5.0	130 up / 100 down	30.0	None
Fiberoptic Laryngoscope					
American Optical LS-7*†	6.4	7.0	120 up / 120 down	50.0	2
Machida FLS-P	4.0	5.5	100 up / 100 down	40.0	1
Fiberoptic Bronchoscopes					
Adult Olympus 4B2	4.9	6.0	180 up / 100 down	59.5	2
Adult Pentax FB15A	4.9	6.0	180 up / 100 down	58.0	2
A-O Scientific Instruments FBS-1	6.0	7.0	150 up / 120 down	60.0	2
Pediatric Olympus BF3C4	3.6	4.5	160 up / 60 down	59.5	1.2
Ultrathin Fiberscope	1.8	3.0		‡	None
Olympus	2.3	3.5		‡	None
	2.4	3.5	None	‡	None
	2.5	3.5		‡	0.5
	2.7	4.0	160 up / 90 down	‡	None

*Battery-powered source also available.
†No photo and video attachment or teaching arm available.
‡Made to customer's specifications.

fibers. The insertion tube should be advanced and withdrawn with the angle section in the neutral position and never with the bending angle knob in the locked position. The knob must not be rotated excessively. No attempt should be made to bend or twist the angle bending section by hand. Twisting the insertion tube too far laterally to manipulate "corners" may result in breakage of fibers.

CLEANING AND STERILIZATION

The instrument must be cleaned and dried thoroughly as soon as possible after use to prevent drying of secretions, blood, mucus, and lubricant on the sheath. The manufacturer's directions for cleaning must be followed if the instrument is to function properly and the warranty remain valid.

The working channel should be cleaned with the brush supplied with the endoscope and air-dried. Brushes are not interchangeable among instruments. Only the insertion tube can be immersed in solution, and no part of the instrument can be steam-autoclaved or boiled. The insertion tube is disinfected by scrubbing with 75% ethyl alcohol or by soaking in 2% glutaraldehyde (Cidex) for 20 minutes.

When ethylene oxide or "gas" sterilization is used, the instrument must be dried prior to sterilization. It is necessary for the endoscope to remain in the aeration chamber a minimum of 12 hours following sterilization. The user must understand the time constraints imposed by ethylene oxide sterilization and schedule use of the instrument accordingly.

ANCILLARY EQUIPMENT

Most difficulties encountered during fiberoptic laryngoscopy relate to maintaining adequate ventilation and anesthesia during the procedure, keeping the endoscope in the midline, and overcoming the obstruction produced by the patient's tongue. These and other problems can usually be managed and the patient's safety insured by utilizing appropriate equipment during endoscopy.

Endoscopic Mask

The Patil-Syracuse mask* was designed to permit laryngoscopy and endotracheal intubation in the anesthetized patient without interfering with ventilation. Administration of oxygen and inhalation anesthesia are continued during the procedure, allowing a longer period for endoscopy while insuring greater patient safety. The fiberoptic laryngoscope can also be used with the mask to identify normal and pathologic airway anatomy in the nonintubated, anesthetized, spontaneously breathing patient.

Endoscopic Oral Airway

The Patil-Syracuse oral airway* prevents the tongue from falling backward and the patient from biting the endoscope. The central groove guides the endoscope in the midline and the slit at the end of the airway permits the tip of the instrument to be directed beyond the epiglottis into the larynx. Lateral channels are provided for suctioning during endoscopy. The airway can be removed without disturbing the position of the endoscope. While ideal in the

---

*Anesthesia Associates, San Marcos, California.

anesthetized patient, the airway is also well tolerated in the sedated patient if adequate topical anesthesia is administered.

Oral Airway with Adapter and Suction Port

Insertion of a right-angle connector with a suction port into a conventional oral airway permits administration of oxygen and inhalation anesthetic agents as well as suctioning during transnasal fiberoptic laryngoscopy.

Binasal Airway

A binasal airway is used for insufflation of oxygen and inhalation anesthetic agents and assisted ventilation during transoral fiberoptic laryngoscopy.

Slit Nasal Airway

A slit catheter or nasal airway facilitates passage of the endoscope through the nose and protects the lens from blood and secretions.

Tongue Retractor

Atraumatic tongue holders and retractors are useful in the patient who has a bulky tongue. Anterior traction on the tongue draws the epiglottis away from the posterior pharyngeal wall and enlarges the area of the oropharynx and hypopharynx.

Bite Block

A bite block should be used to protect the endoscope in the awake patient.

Atomizer for Topical Anesthesia

Several types of atomizers are available for application of topical laryngotracheal anesthesia. The McIntosh laryngeal spray offers the advantage of an adjustable tip.

Laryngeal Forceps

The Jackson laryngeal forceps are designed specifically for applying local anesthetic agents to the piriform fossae.

Defogging Agent

A soap product or pHisoHex must be used to defog the lens of the endoscope. Reapplication is necessary if the endoscopy is prolonged.

Cricothyrotomy Needle

A large-bore intravenous (IV) catheter can be used. Insertion of a 3-mm endotracheal tube adapter into the hub of the catheter permits attachment to an anesthetic circuit or Ambu bag.

AVAILABLE INSTRUMENTATION

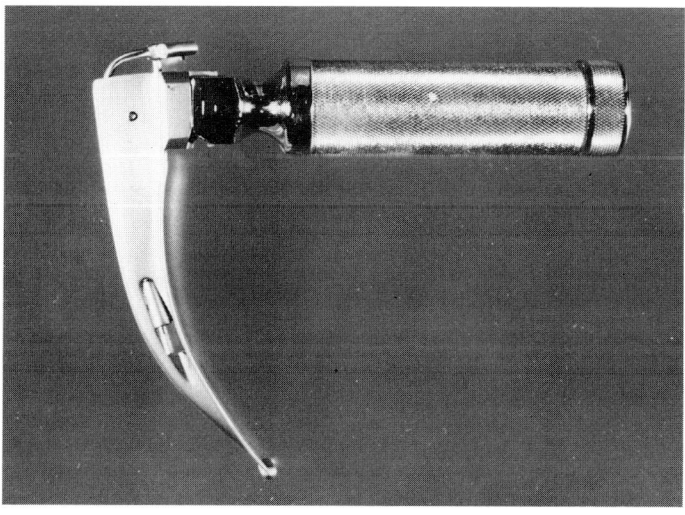

Fig 2–1.—A laryngoscope with a fiberoptic light source offers the advantages of bright, continuous light. It is especially useful when laryngoscopy is prolonged.

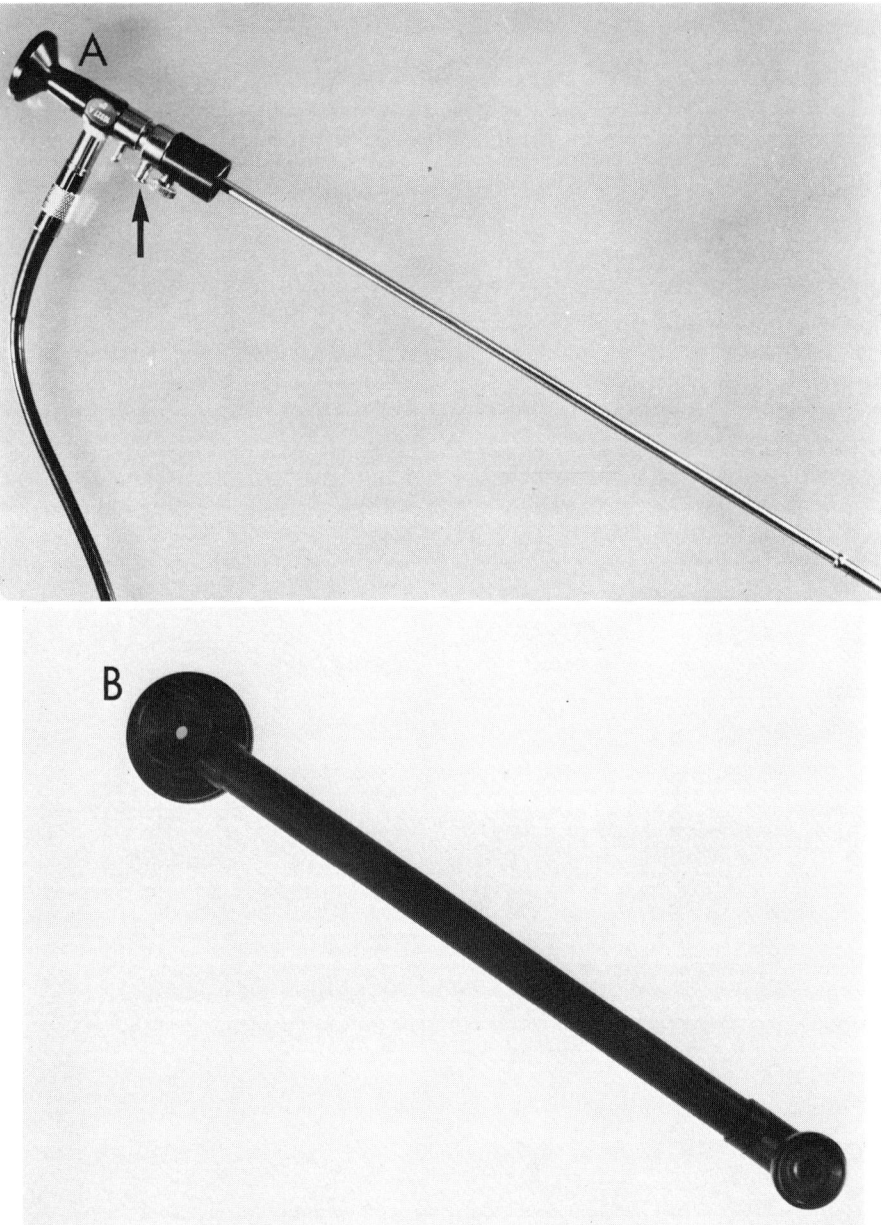

Fig 2–2.—**A,** the Stortz optical stylet, a rigid instrument available in pediatric and adult sizes, is used for examination of the larynx and endotracheal intubation. A curved laryngoscope blade is utilized to retract the tongue before introduction of the optical stylet. The *arrow* identifies the port on the external sheath through which oxygen can be insufflated, local anesthesia instilled, or secretions suctioned. **B,** teaching attachment.

INSTRUMENTATION AND AUXILIARY EQUIPMENT

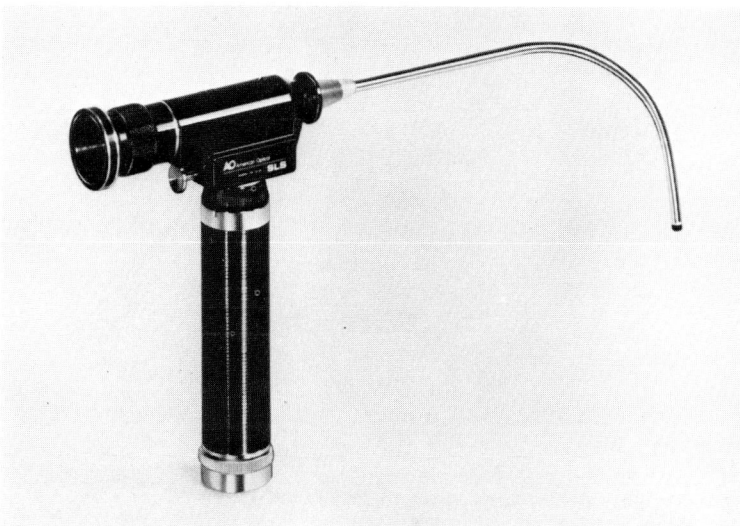

Fig 2–3.—The curve of the insertion tube of the semirigid American Optical fiberoptic stylet must be established prior to introduction into the patient, since it cannot be altered unless the instrument is withdrawn. The distal 2.5 cm is rigid.

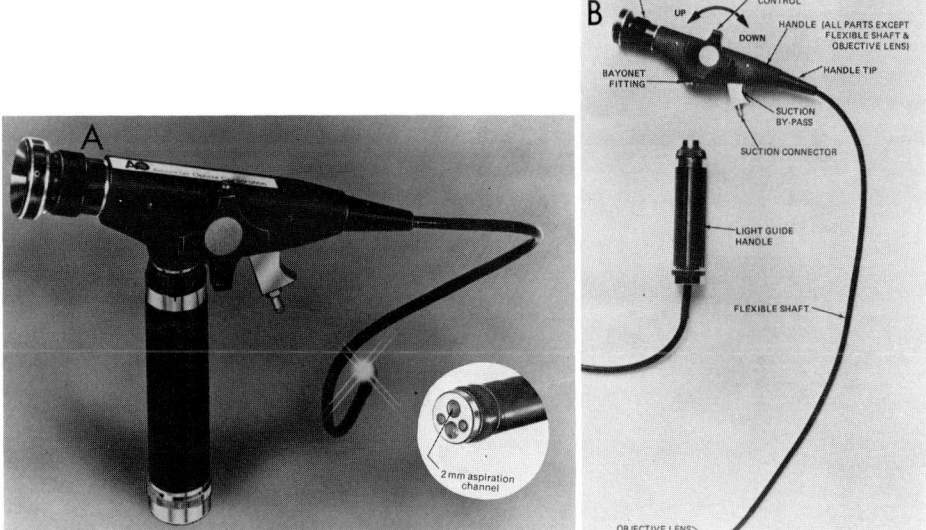

Fig 2–4.—**A,** The American Optical fiberoptic laryngoscope with aspiration channel. **B,** The components of the instrument.

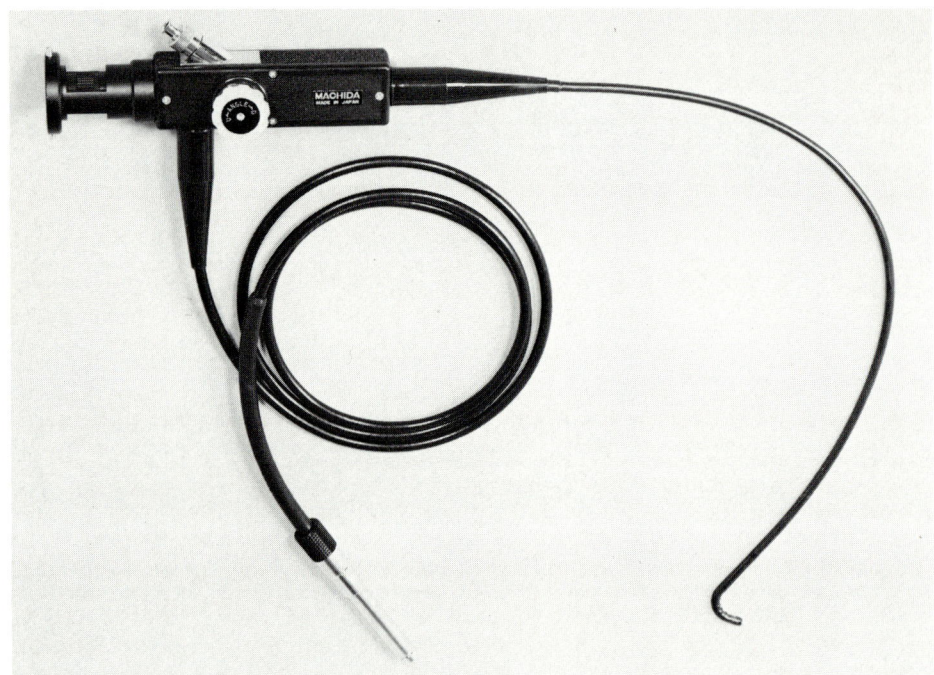

Fig 2–5.—The Machida fiberoptic laryngoscope.

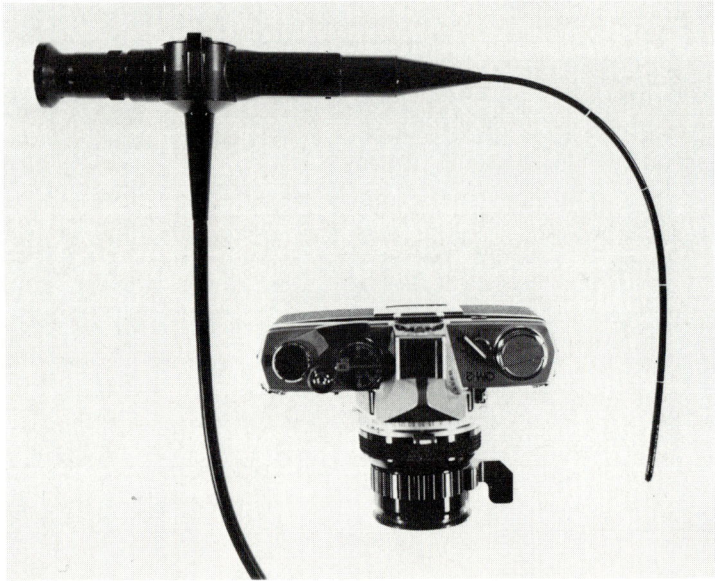

Fig 2–6.—The Olympus fiberoptic rhinolaryngoscope with camera attachment. The insertion tube is shorter than that of an adult bronchoscope and longer than that of an adult laryngoscope. There is no suction port.

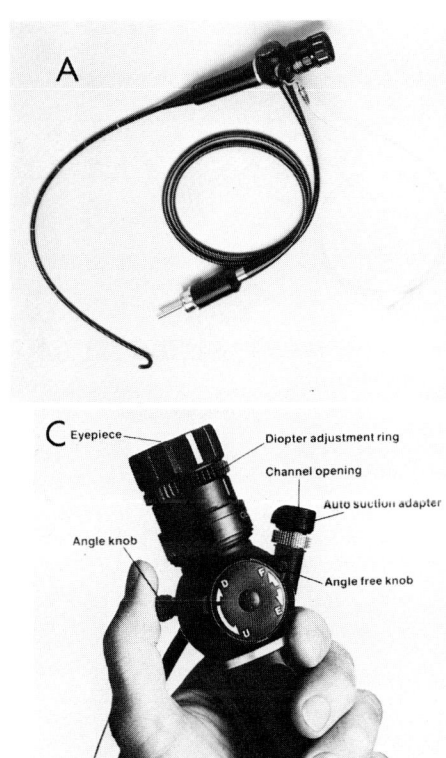
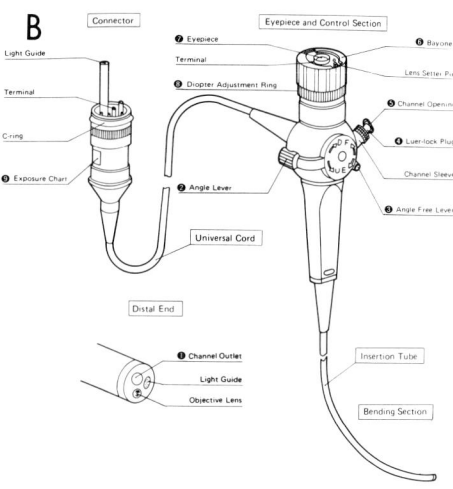

Fig 2-7.—A, Olympus pediatric fiberoptic bronchoscope with tubing attached for insufflation of oxygen or suctioning. **B,** components of the instrument. **C,** control section.

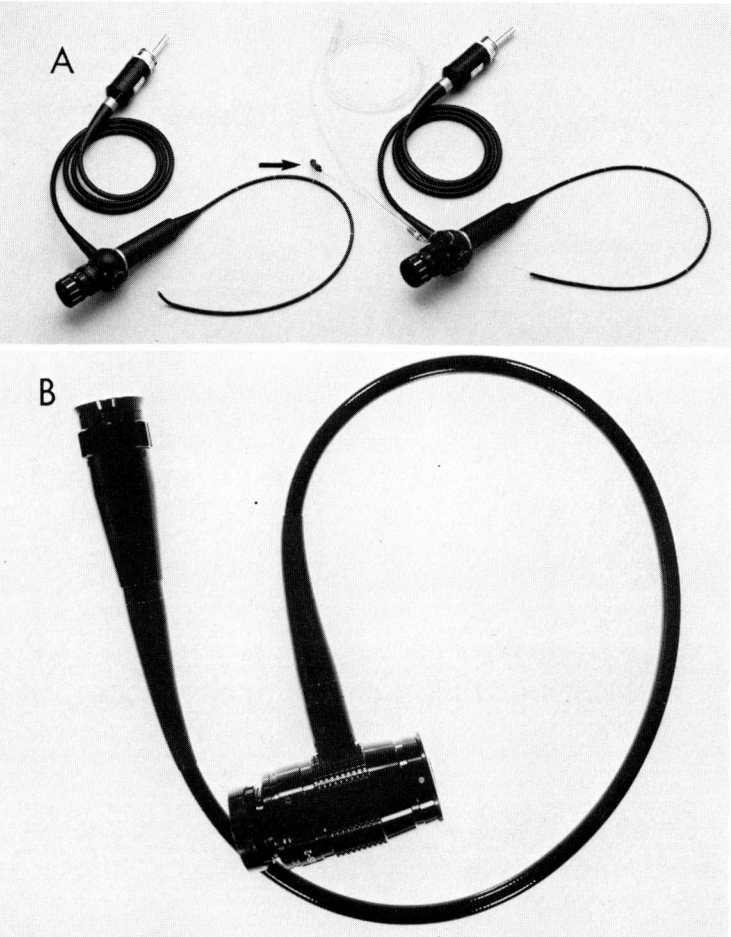

Fig 2–8.—A, Olympus adult fiberoptic bronchoscopes. The *arrow* indicates a cleaning wire within the biopsy channel and extending through the end of the insertion tube. **B,** teaching attachment.

INSTRUMENTATION AND AUXILIARY EQUIPMENT 19

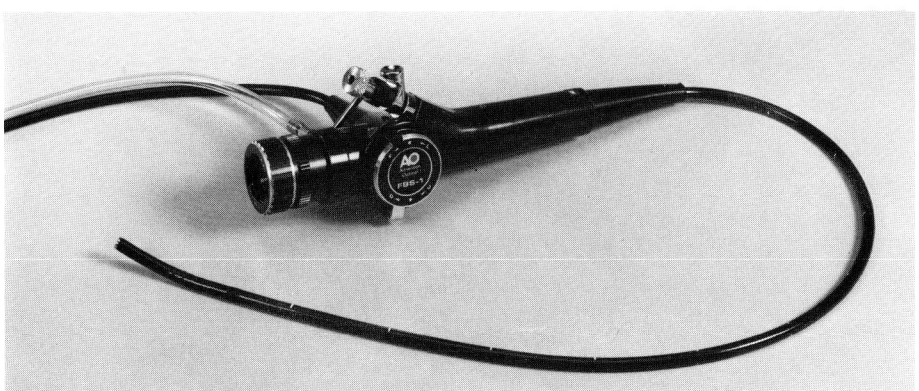

Fig 2–9.—A–O Scientific Instruments fiberoptic adult bronchoscope with suction and operating channels.

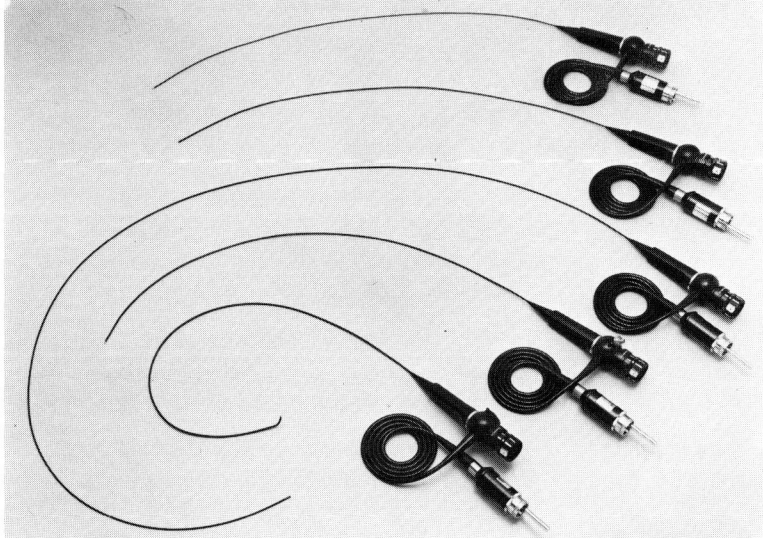

Fig 2–10.—Olympus Ultrathin fiberscopes. The 2.5-mm model has a suction channel and the 2.7-mm model has a bending angle.

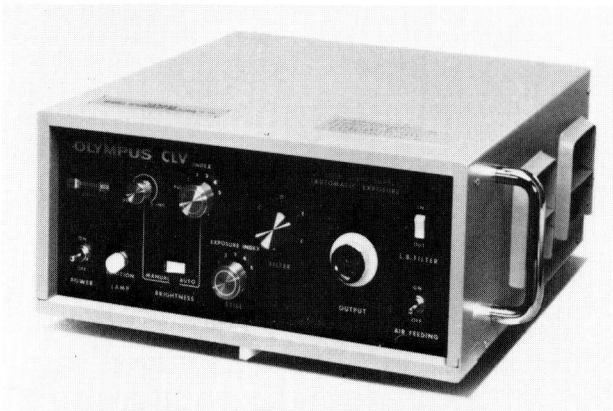

Fig 2–11.—Light source for fiberoptic endoscopes.

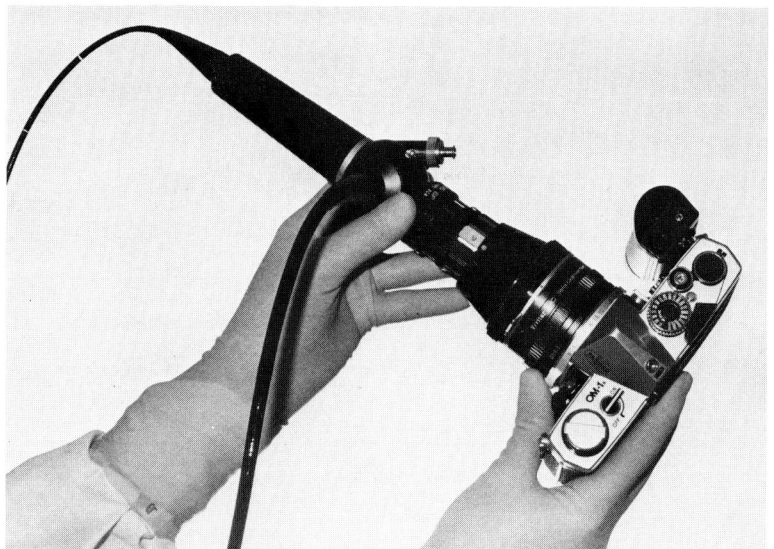

Fig 2–12.—A 35-mm camera with adapter used with Olympus fiberoptic endoscope.

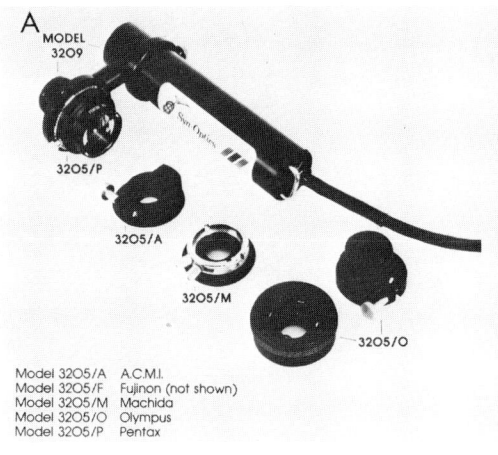
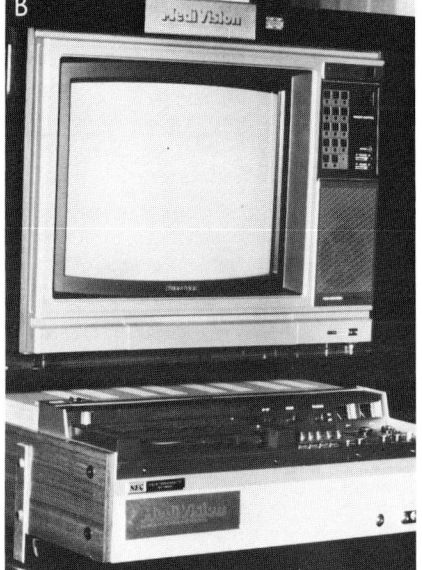

Fig 2–13.—Video camera with endoscope attachment **(A)** for transmission of image to television screen **(B)**.

CARE OF THE INSTRUMENT

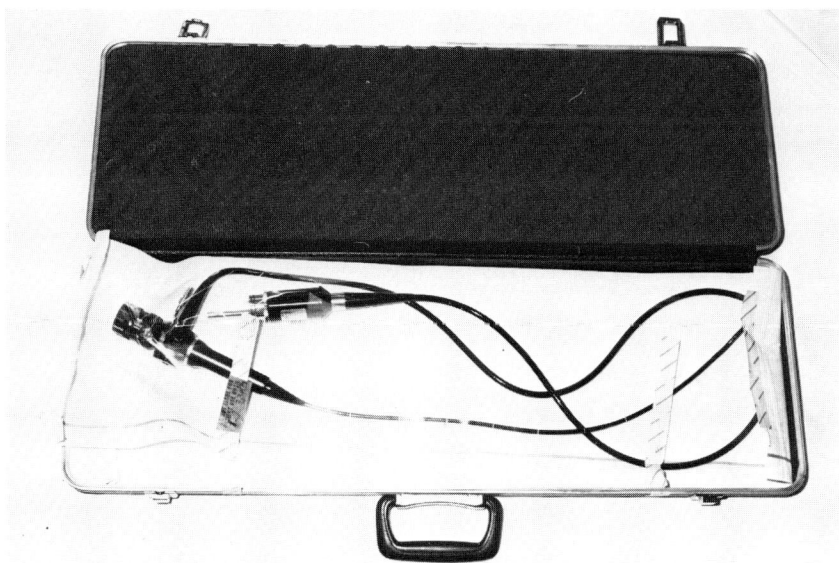

Fig 2–14.—Gas-sterilized fiberoptic endoscope in padded case. Special attention must be given to avoid kinking the insertion tube during packaging. A transparent wrapper is used to call attention to the nature and delicacy of the instrument during loading of the autoclave and subsequent handling.

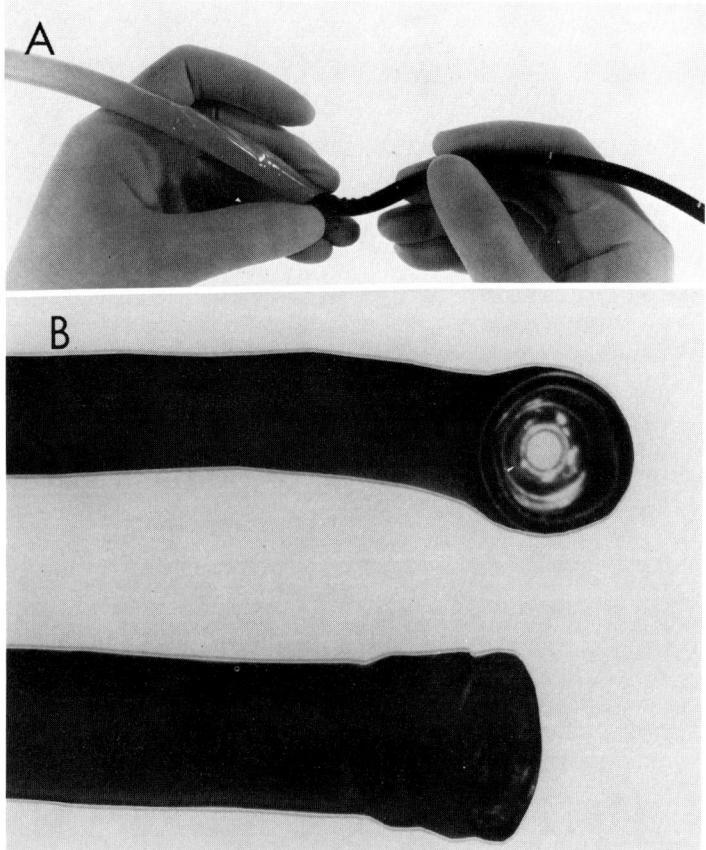

Fig 2–15.—**A,** Forcing the endoscope through a small ETT may result in damage to the fibers or angle bend mechanism. **B,** The outer sheath of the insertion tube may be herniated over the lens as a result of insufficient lubrication or forcing the insertion tube into an ETT that is too small.

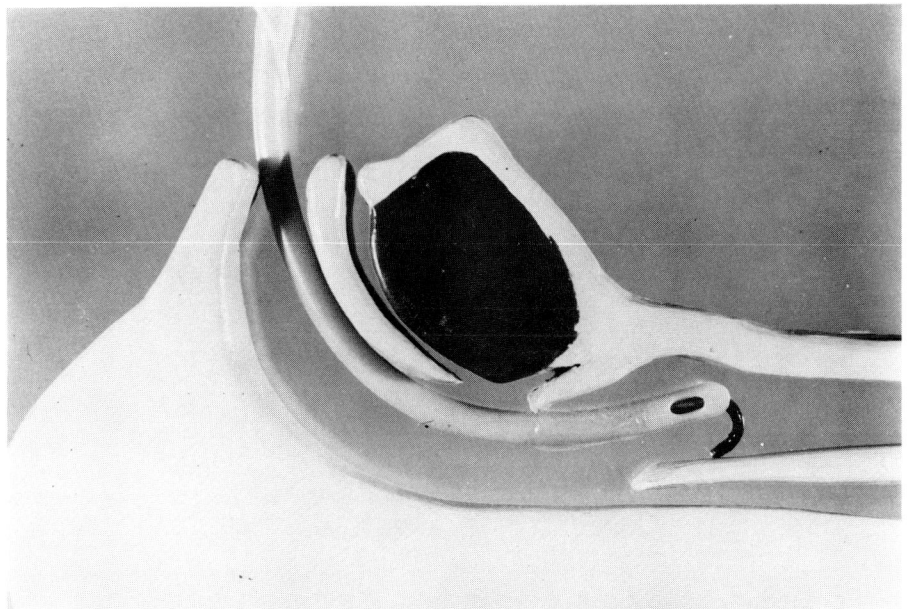

Fig 2–16.—The insertion tube must not be withdrawn or advanced with the distal tip angled as shown.

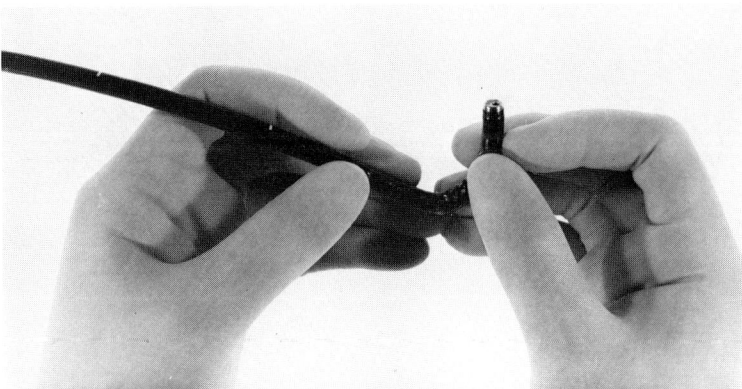

Fig 2–17.—The angle bend tip must not be manipulated by hand.

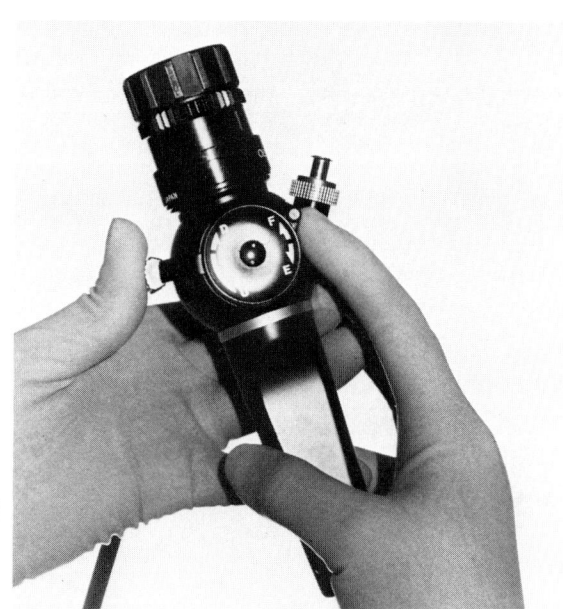

Fig 2–18.—The angle bend knob should be kept in the free position **(F)** rather than engaged **(E)** during any manipulation of the fiberoptic endoscope to avoid damage to fibers and to the angle bend mechanism.

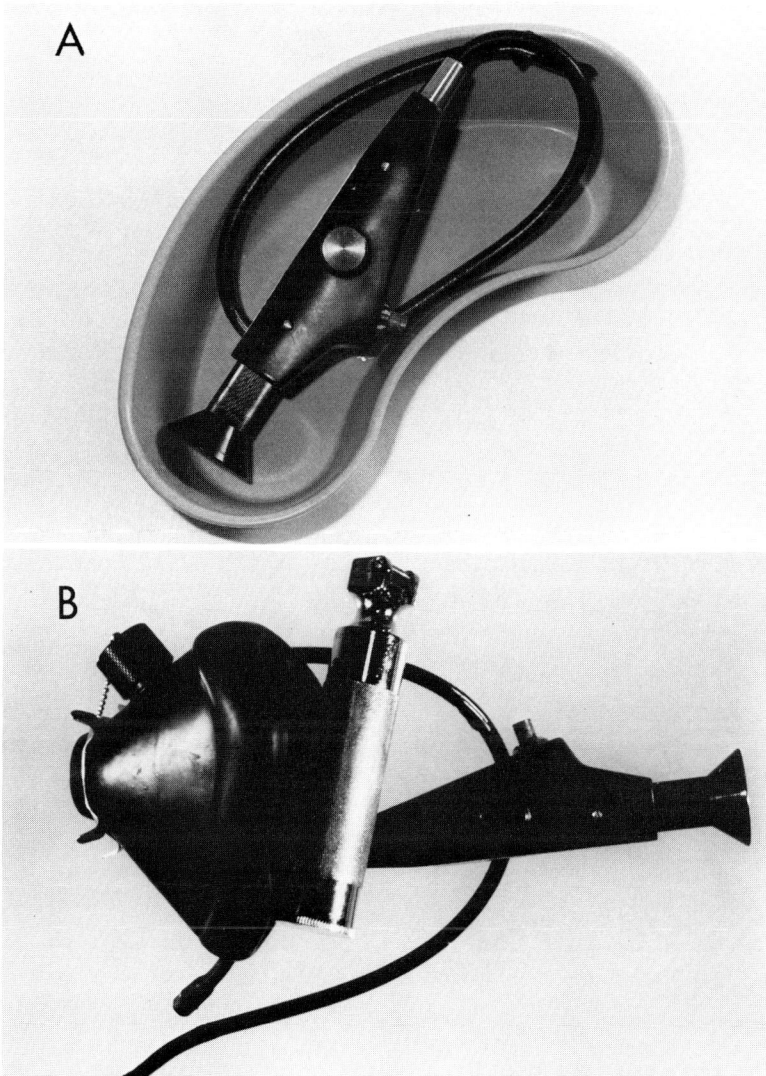

Fig 2–19.—Following use of the instrument, care must be taken to avoid sharply coiling the insertion tube **(A)** or placing other equipment on it **(B)**.

CLEANING AND STERILIZATION

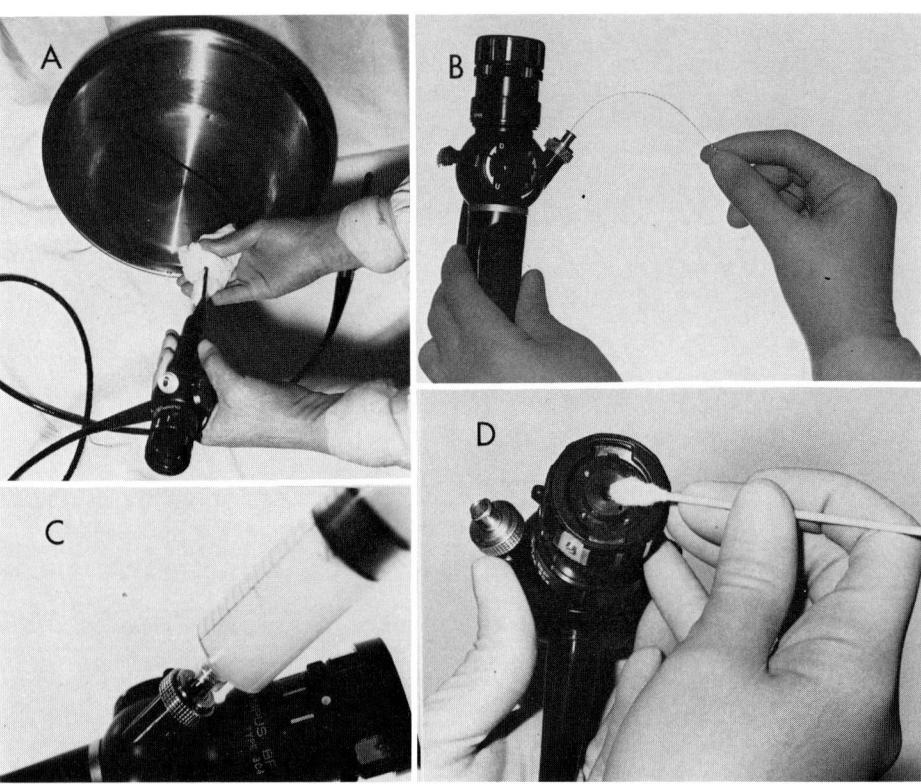

Fig 2–20.—**A,** The sheath of the insertion tube should be cleaned with water immediately after use. Only the insertion tube can be immersed. **B,** The operating channel is to be cleaned only with the brush provided with the endoscope, since brushes are not interchangeable among instruments. **C,** The operating channel is thoroughly flushed with water and air-dried before gas sterilization. **D,** The proximal lens may be cleaned with 75% alcohol using a cotton swab.

INSTRUMENTATION AND AUXILIARY EQUIPMENT

ANCILLARY EQUIPMENT

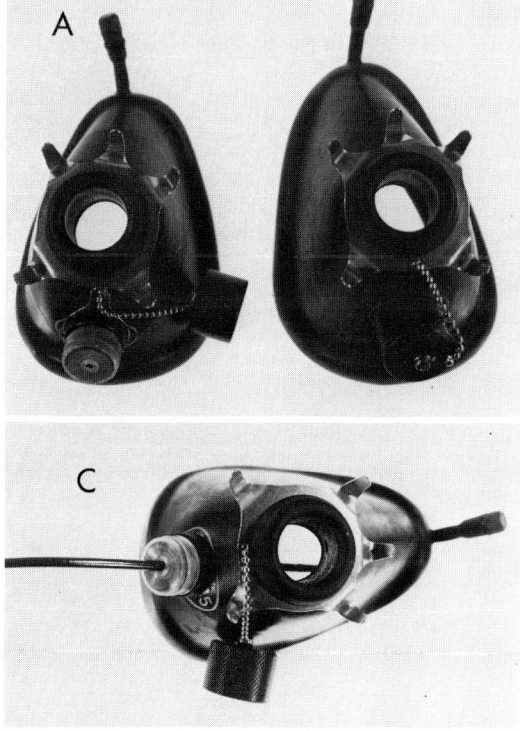
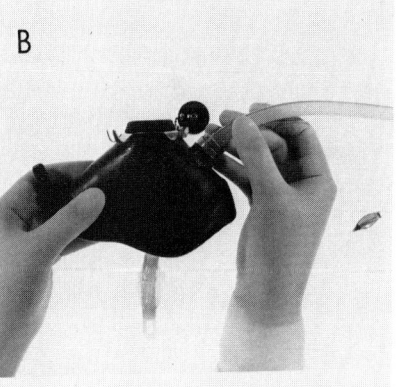

Fig 2–21.—**A,** the Patil-Syracuse endoscopic mask with endoscopic port. **B,** an 8.5-mm ETT inserted through the endoscopic port of the Patil-Syracuse mask. **C,** the construction of the diaphragm on the endoscopic port provides an airtight seal with the smallest of pediatric bronchoscopes currently available.

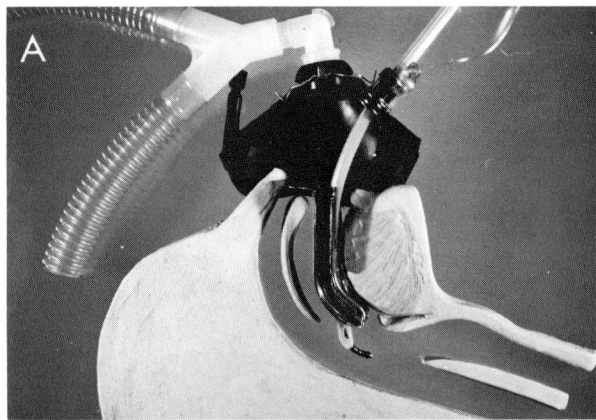

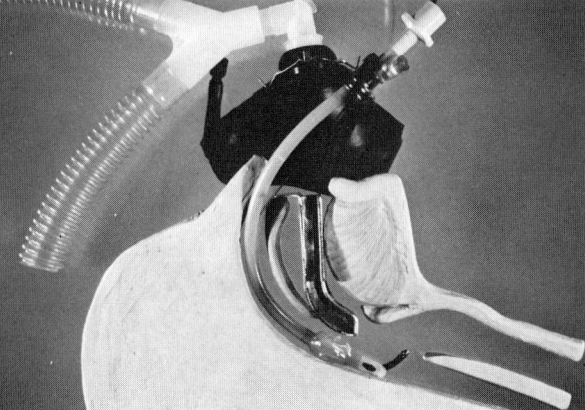

Fig 2–22.—**Top,** cross section of the Patil-Syracuse mask showing orotracheal intubation utilizing the endoscopic port. **Bottom,** cross section of the Patil-Syracuse mask showing nasotracheal intubation utilizing the endoscopic port.

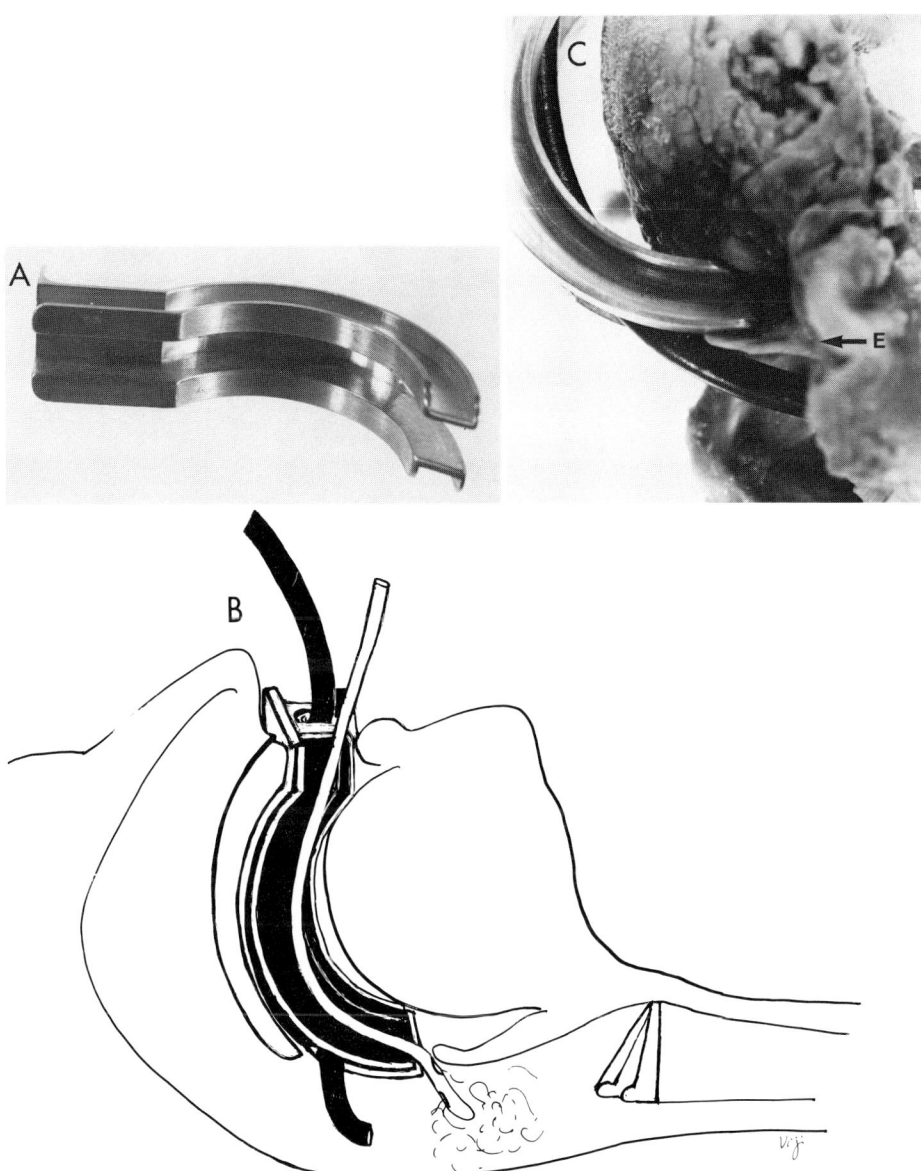

Fig 2–23.—**A,** The Patil-Syracuse airway has a central groove, lateral suction channels, and a distal slit. **B,** The central groove maintains the midline position of the insertion tube. Suctioning is performed through the side channels. **C,** The slit at the end of the airway permits the insertion tube to be introduced beyond the epiglottis *(E)*. The papillae of the tongue appear disproportionately prominent as a result of magnification.

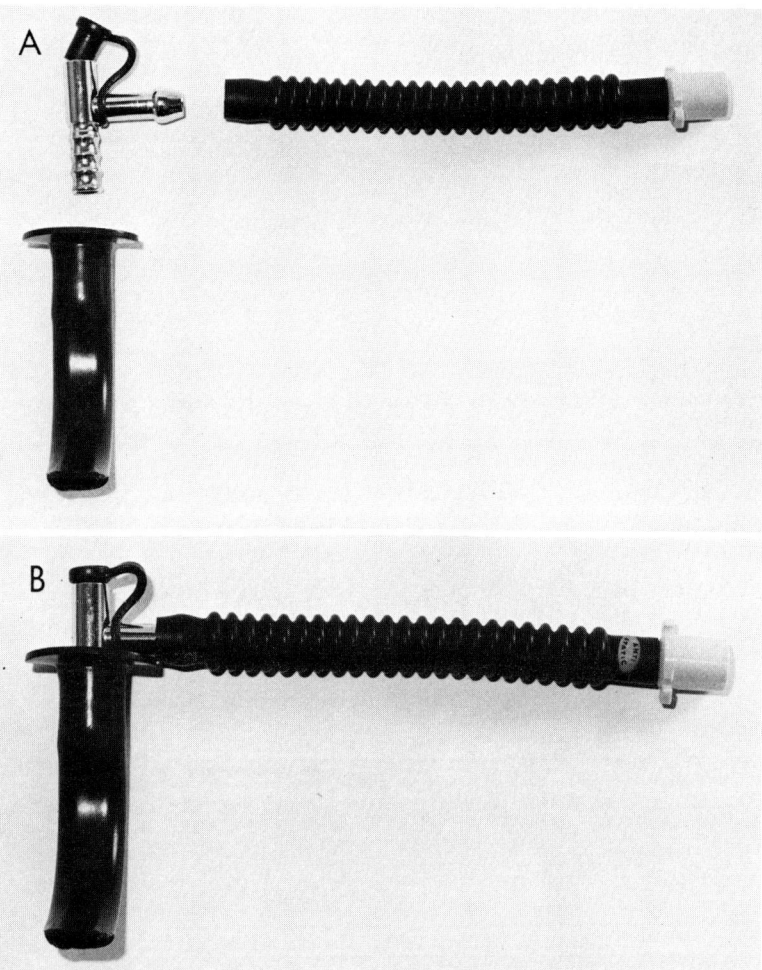

Fig 2–24.—Right-angle connector with a suction port is inserted into a conventional oral airway for use during transnasal fiberoptic laryngoscopy. **A,** components; **B,** assembled.

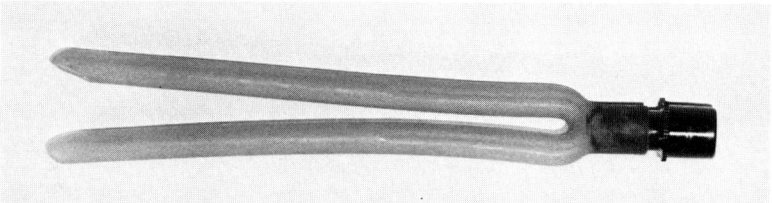

Fig 2–25.—A binasal airway used to administer anesthesia or oxygen during orotracheal endoscopic intubation.

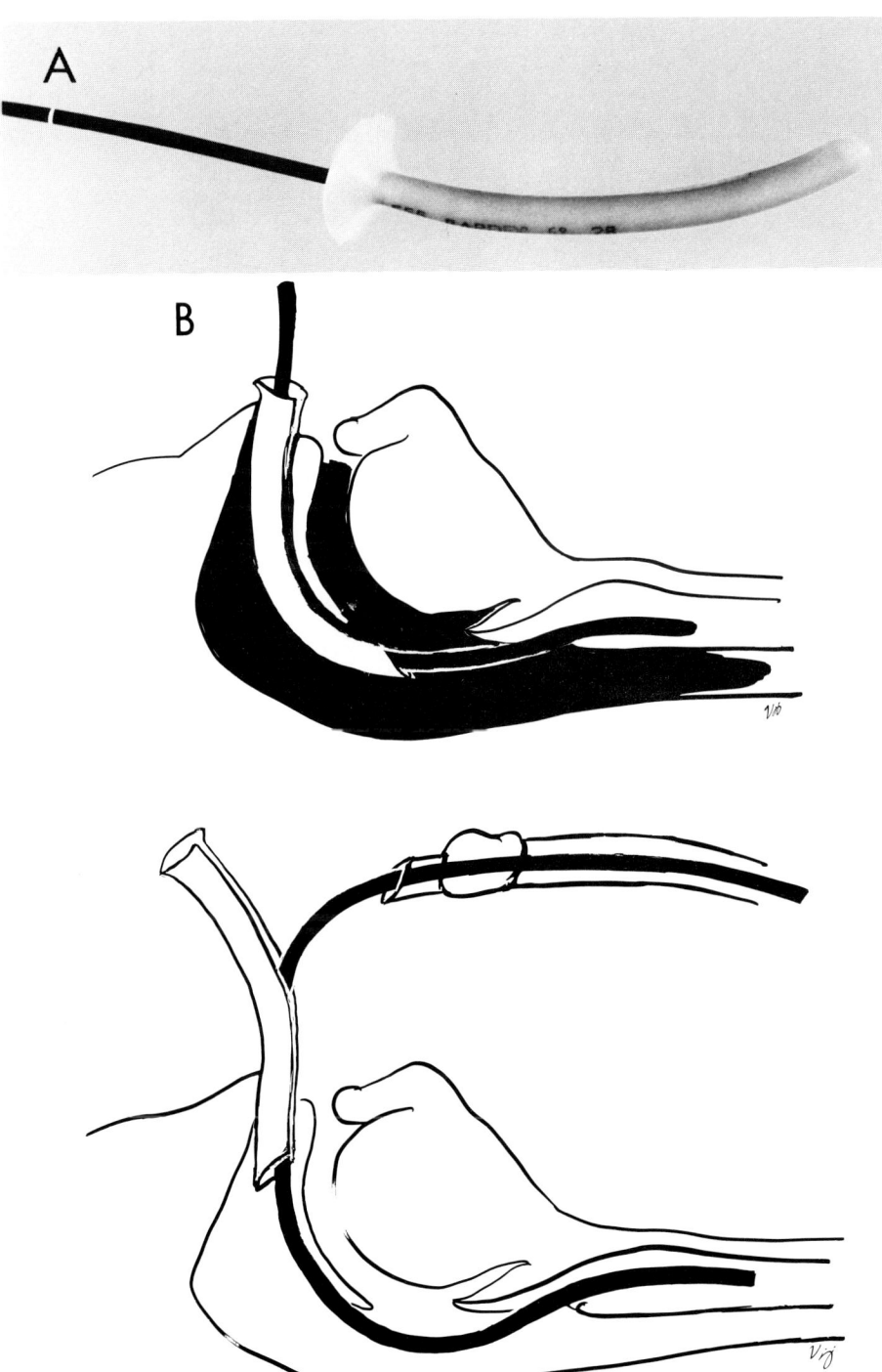

Fig 2–26.—**(A)** Tissue trauma is minimized and placement of the insertion tube is facilitated if the latter is threaded into a nasal airway prior to passage. The airway should be slit longitudinally before insertion of the instrument to permit removal of the airway without altering the position of the insertion tube. The tip of the insertion tube must not protrude through the end of the airway when passed through the nose. This technique is especially useful when using a pediatric bronchoscope because of the delicacy of the instrument **(B).**

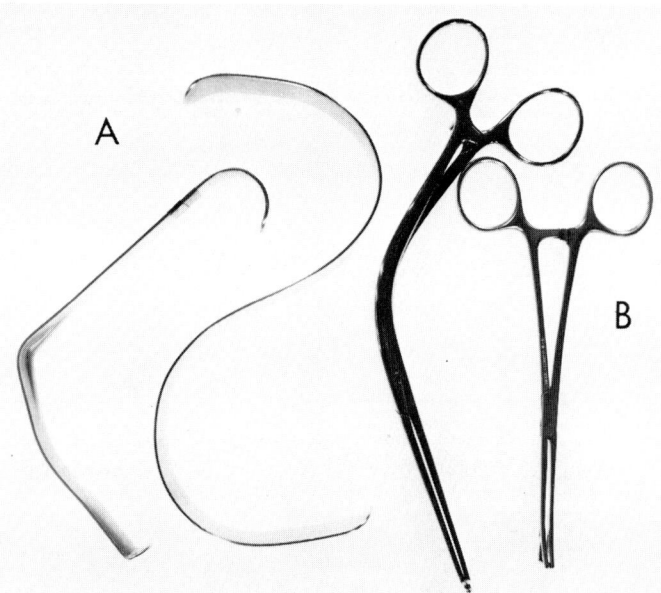

Fig 2–27.—Malleable tongue retractors **(A)** and atraumatic tongue holders **(B)** used to facilitate endoscopy.

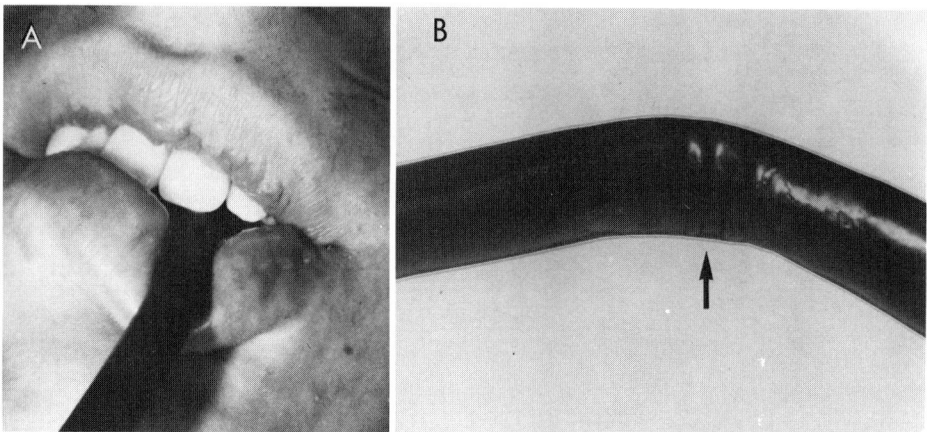

Fig 2–28.—A patient biting the insertion tube **(A)** resulting in damage to the instrument **(B)**.

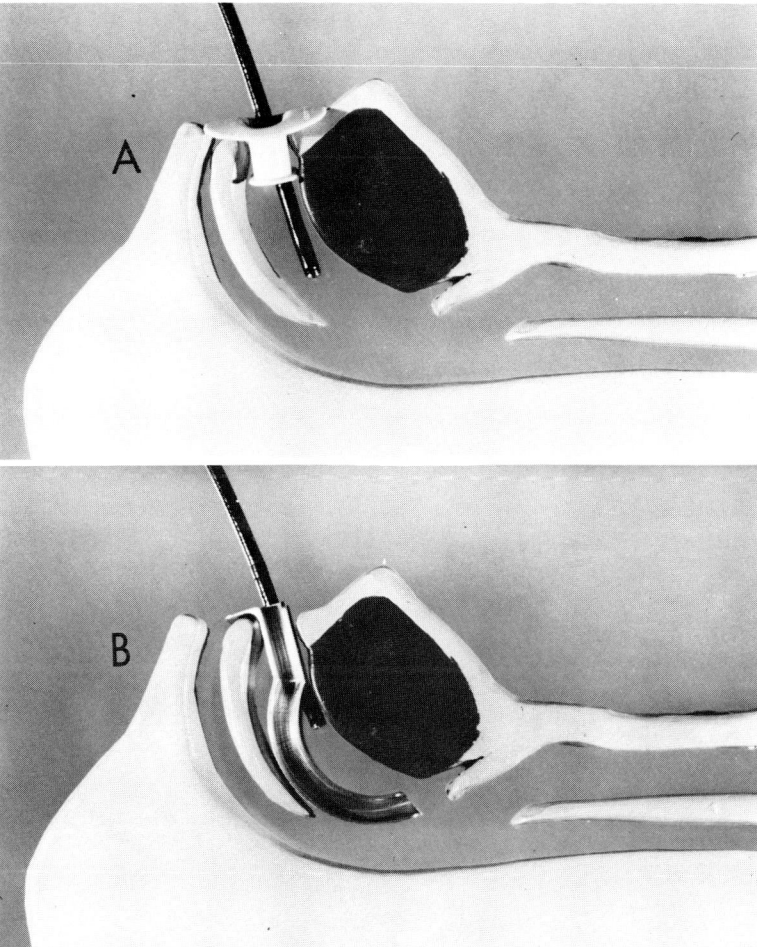

Fig 2–29.—Plastic bite block **(A)** and metal airway **(B)** used to prevent patient's biting the insertion tube.

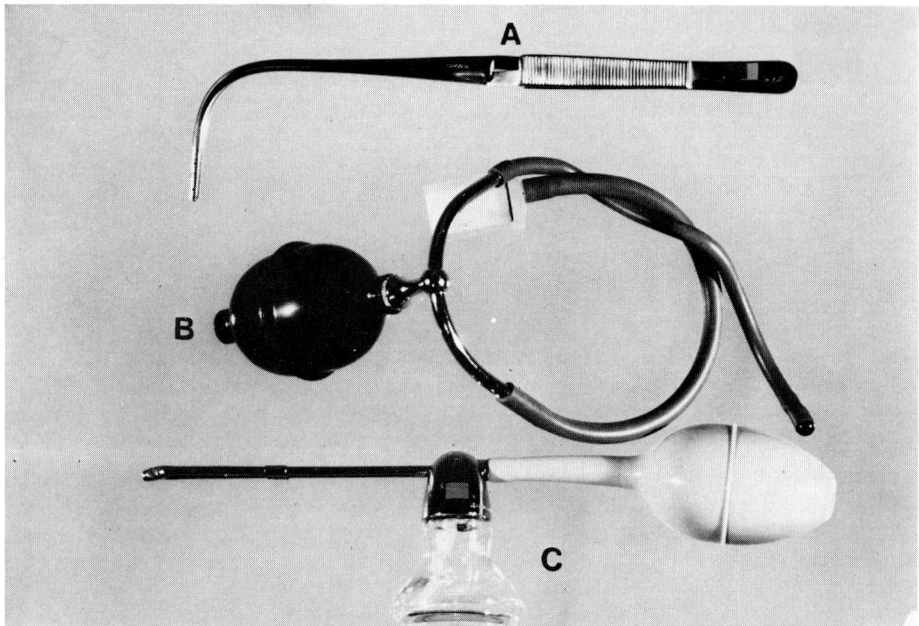

Fig 2–30.—**A,** laryngeal forceps used to hold sponge saturated with local anesthetic when anesthetizing the internal laryngeal nerve in the piriform fossa. **B,** laryngeal atomizer with adjustable tip for instillation of local anesthesia. **C,** Macintosh spray with flexible tip to anesthetize the oral cavity and larynx.

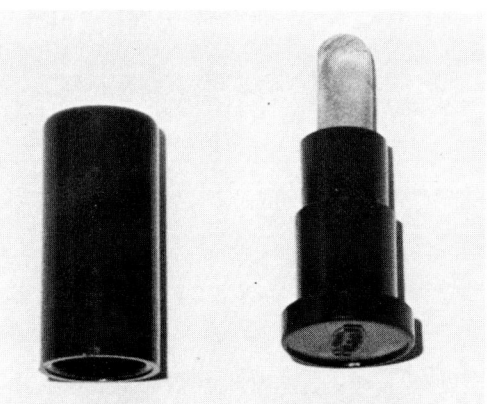

Fig 2–31.—Defogging soap should always be applied before focusing the lens. pHisoHex may also be used.

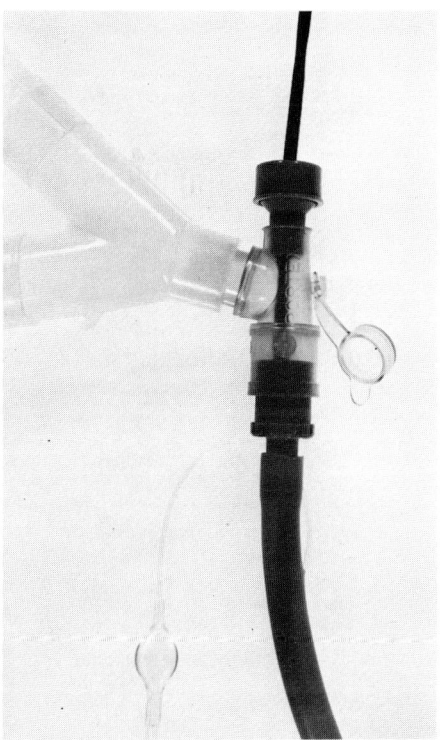

Fig 2–32.—Endoscopic adapter with port for insertion tube is used in the intubated patient.

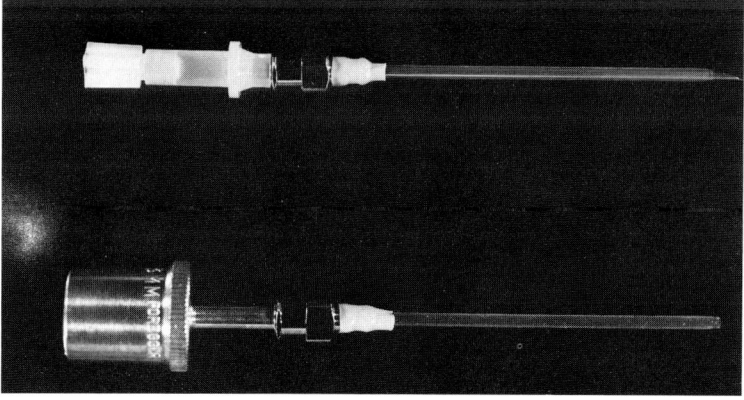

Fig 2–33.—A large-bore IV catheter can be used for cricothyrotomy in an emergency. Use of a 3-mm ETT connector in the hub of the catheter permits attachment to an anesthetic circuit or Ambu bag.

3 / Pharmacology of Adjuvant Drugs

THE ANESTHETIC TECHNIQUE must be chosen on the basis of the patient's physical status, airway anatomy, and the indications for endoscopy. Factors such as recent ingestion of food, drug allergy, and patient preference must be considered.

ANTISIALAGOGUES

Unless contraindicated by concomitant disease, antisialagogues should be administered preoperatively when fiberoptic laryngoscopy is planned. Although the time of onset and duration of action of the drugs vary, the drying effects of atropine, scopolamine, and glycopyrrolate are usually manifest within 10–15 minutes of intramuscular (IM) administration. The action of glycopyrrolate lasts up to 7 hours, whereas the effects of the belladonna alkaloids are usually dissipated within 4 hours. The drying effects of the drugs are less predictable when they are administered intravenously (IV).

VASOCONSTRICTORS

A topical vasoconstrictor should be applied prior to passing an endotracheal tube or endoscope through the nose to lessen the possibility of obscuring the lens with blood. Cocaine provides profound anesthesia, constricts blood vessels, and shrinks swollen mucosal membranes. Tachycardia usually occurs as a result of increased central sympathetic stimulation and interference with the uptake of norepinephrine by adrenergic nerve terminals. Phenylephrine (Neo-Synephrine), also a potent vasoconstrictor, exerts virtually no systemic effects when a few drops of 0.25%–0.5% solution are applied to the nasal mucosa.

GENERAL ANESTHESIA

No alteration of technique is required to induce general anesthesia in patients scheduled for fiberoptic laryngoscopy who have normal airway anatomy and have received nothing by mouth for an appropriate period. It is, however, advisable to increase the inspired oxygen concentration ($F_{I_{O_2}}$) prior to endoscopy. The effect of $F_{I_{O_2}}$ in the apneic patient is shown in Figure 3–1.

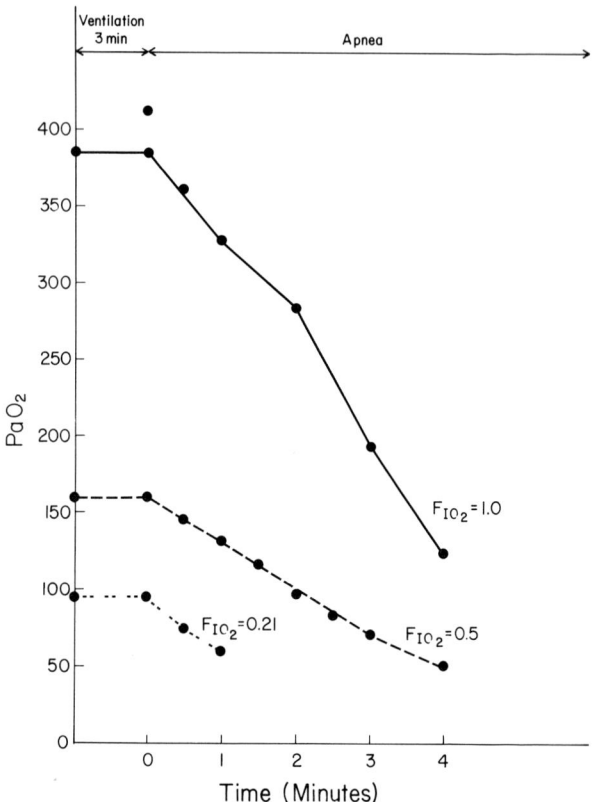

Fig 3–1.—The rate of desaturation of arterial blood in apneic patients following ventilation with varying inspired oxygen concentrations. (Modified from Heller M.L., Watson T.R.: Polarographic study of arterial oxygenation during apnea in man. *N. Engl. J. Med.* 264:326, 1961.)

Among the factors producing distortion of the airway and necessitating placement of the endotracheal tube prior to induction of general anesthesia are congenital malformations, trauma, tumors, previous surgical procedures, and burn scar contractures. The anesthesiologist's preoperative evaluation of such patients must include a review of previous anesthetic experiences and consultation with the surgeon. Indirect laryngoscopy may be indicated and can be performed by the anesthesiologist as well as the surgeon (Fig 3–2). Radiologic examinations that may be useful in assessing the airway include x-rays and fluoroscopy of the neck and chest, tomograms, and computerized tomographic (CT) scans.

An inhalation induction is appropriate for some patients when difficulty with endoscopy and intubation is anticipated but mask ventilation poses no problem. Sedatives, hypnotics, and narcotics are omitted or administered in small, incremental doses, and muscle relaxants are avoided prior to laryngoscopy. A competent surgeon, rigid bronchoscopes, functional light sources, tracheostomy set, and cricothyrotomy needle must be available for early intervention if airway obstruction occurs.

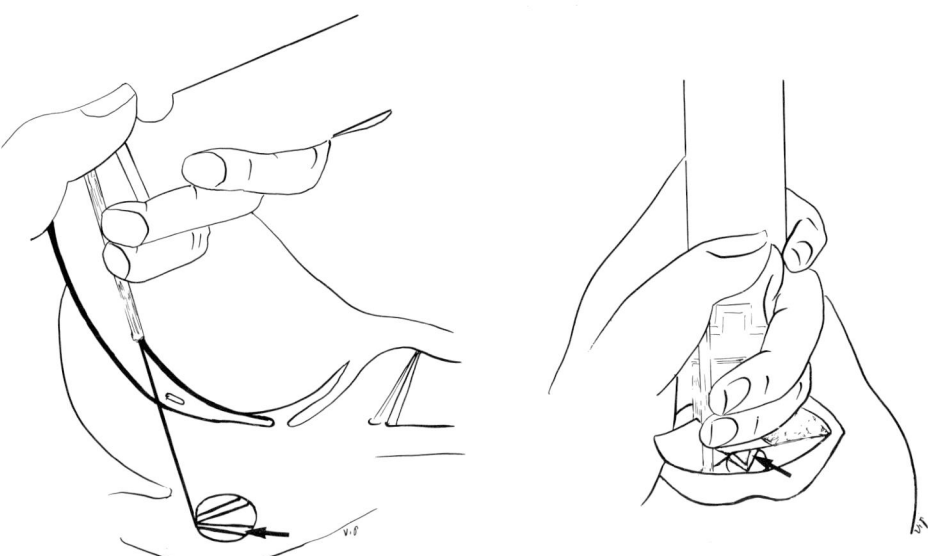

Fig 3–2.—The airway is assessed by indirect laryngoscopy preoperatively utilizing a dental mirror and curved laryngoscope blade.

Halothane is the least pungent of the volatile agents, making it preferable to enflurane or isoflurane. However, if topical cocaine or epinephrine-containing solutions are used concomitantly, the potential for cardiac arrhythmias is greatest with halothane. The concentration of volatile agents must be increased slowly to prevent coughing and laryngospasm. The decision to use nitrous oxide is dependent on the patient's airway pathology. Many anesthesiologists omit the agent entirely to provide a higher inspired oxygen concentration; others use it in selected patients. Laryngoscopy should not be attempted until the patient is deeply anesthetized and is best performed utilizing an endoscopic airway and a mask with an endoscopic adapter. An assistant should monitor the patient while the primary anesthesiologist is performing the laryngoscopy, since it is easy for the endoscopist to become so involved in the procedure that he is oblivious to indications of patient instability.

LOCAL ANESTHESIA

Local anesthetic agents may be applied topically, infiltrated or instilled. Adequate analgesia can be provided safely if the anesthesiologist does not exceed recommended drug dosages (Table 3–1) and allows sufficient time for the agents to take effect prior to laryngoscopy. Absorption of local anesthetics from mucous membranes is extremely rapid. When refillable atomizers are used, the

TABLE 3–1.—LOCAL ANESTHETIC AGENTS

AGENT	CONCENTRATION (%)	CLINICAL USE	MAXIMUM DOSE (mg/kg)	Total mg
Cocaine	4	Topical	3–4	200
Lidocaine (Xylocaine)	2–4	Topical	4	200
	1–2	Infiltration	7	500
Tetracaine (Pontocaine)	0.25–1	Topical	1–2	100
Mepivacaine (Carbocaine)	1–2	Infiltration	7	500
Bupivcaine (Marcaine, Sensorcaine)	0.25–0.50	Infiltration	2–3	200
Etidocaine (Duranest)	0.5	Infiltration	4–5	400
Benzocaine ⎱ (Cetacaine)	14			
Tetracaine ⎰	2	Topical	*	*

*Spraying in excess of 2 seconds not recommended.

maximum safe dosage should be calculated and only that amount placed in the unit. It is especially easy to overdose a patient when prefilled multidose containers are employed. Because the amounts of drug dispensed vary, the supplier's instructions must be read and carefully followed. Standard resuscitation equipment and medications for treating toxic reactions must be readily available.

INTRAVENOUS SEDATION

Narcotics and tranquilizers can be used alone or in combination for most patients in whom laryngoscopy is performed with topical anesthesia. Agents with the shortest duration of action are preferable so that the patient will be able to protect his airway on termination of the procedure. Because patient responses are so variable, the drugs are best administered IV in the operating room and dosages precisely titrated. The major side effects of the narcotics are respiratory depression and chest wall rigidity.

Although initially very popular for sedation during endoscopic procedures, Innovar has several drawbacks. It is a fixed combination preparation (1 ml = 0.05 mg fentanyl citrate and 2.5 mg droperidol), and the components are very different in duration of action. Sedation may persist for more than 24 hours and extrapyramidal movements are often delayed for 6–12 hours. Decreased laryngeal competence, patient refusal of surgery, and intense anxiety despite apparent calmness have been observed following administration of the drug.

Diazepam is probably the most frequently employed agent. A major advantage is the anterograde amnesia experienced by many patients. The dosage varies greatly: unconsciousness is produced following IV injection of 5 mg/70 kg in some patients; others do not become drowsy until up to 1 mg/kg of the drug is administered. There is a correlation between the degree of ventilatory depression and the state of consciousness. Ventilatory depression may be evident within one minute of injection and persist a half hour or longer. Ventilation is more depressed in the absence of stimulation; thus, a patient who is ventilating adequately in the immediate postoperative period may hypoventilate when removed from the stimulating environment of the operating and recovery areas. Concurrent administration of narcotics augments the ventilatory depression of diazepam.

4 / Anatomy for the Endoscopist

THE ANESTHESIOLOGIST accustomed to direct laryngoscopy will find that the perspective is entirely different when anatomical structures are viewed through the fiberoptic endoscope. To become adept at fiberoptic laryngoscopy, the anesthesiologist must first learn to identify normal structures by studying endoscopic photographs, descriptive drawings, and anatomical models.

Even with appropriate preparation, the anesthesiologist will notice several differences when first performing fiberoptic endoscopy on patients: the size of the image is different, some structures are actively moving and others are abnormally lax. Fogging of the lens and distortion of the image by secretions are inevitable. However, the anesthesiologist who has taken the time to thoroughly learn the anatomy of the upper airway will be able to recognize familiar structures and identify deviations from normal.

The position of the tongue, a highly muscular structure, may make passage of the endoscope impossible and preclude endotracheal intubation. Altering the position of the head, manipulating the jaw, and retracting the tongue change the configuration of the pharynx and the relation of the larynx to other anatomical structures.

It is essential that the anesthesiologist be familiar with the innervation of the airway and normal anatomy prior to attempting fiberoptic endoscopy.

Normal anatomical structures are shown in the accompanying endoscopic photographs and drawings. Numerous anatomical variants are illustrated in chapter 6.

SENSORY INNERVATION OF THE AIRWAY

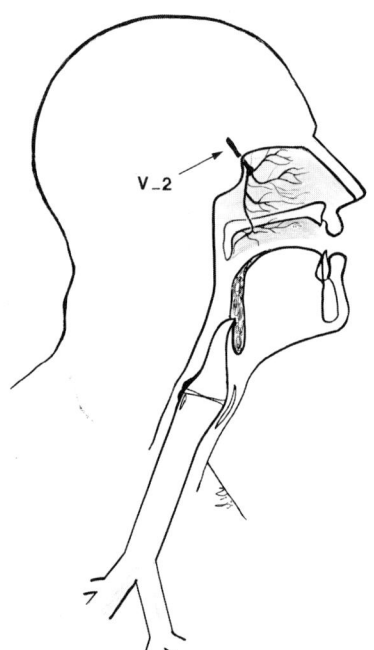

Fig 4–1.—Structures innervated by the maxillary branch (V-2) of the trigeminal nerve include: upper teeth and gums, vestibule of the nose, upper lip, nasal cavity, palate, and the anterior roof of the pharynx.

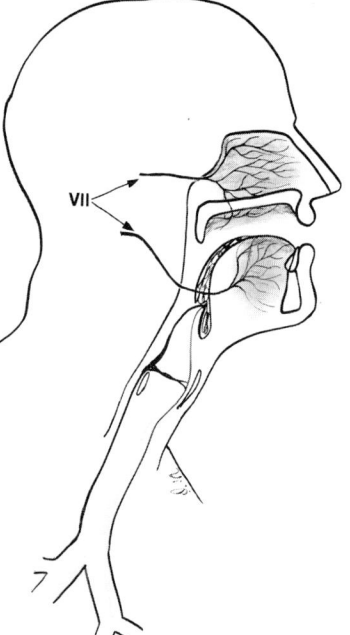

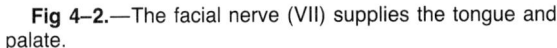

Fig 4–2.—The facial nerve (VII) supplies the tongue and palate.

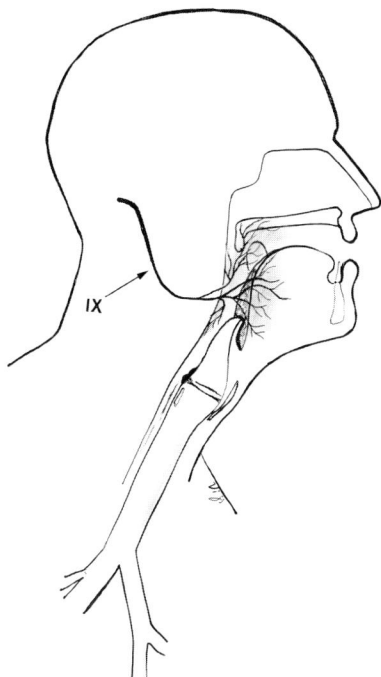

Fig 4–3.—Structures innervated by the glossopharyngeal nerve (IX) include: the pharyngeal wall, oropharyngeal isthmus, undersurface of the soft palate, tonsils, pharyngeal arches, posterior third of the tongue, and roof of the pharynx.

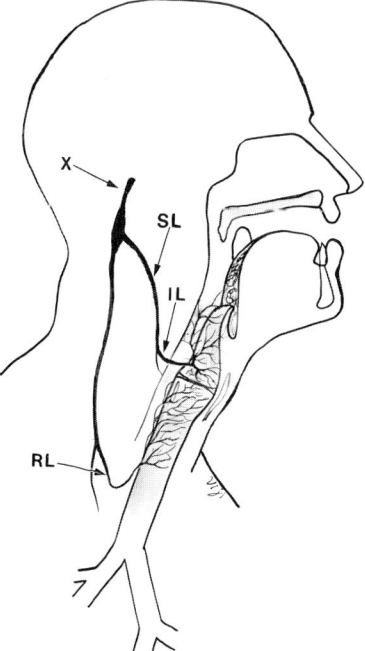

Fig 4–4.—Sensory distribution of the vagus nerve (X): The internal laryngeal nerve (IL), which is a branch of the superior laryngeal nerve (SL), supplies the larynx above the vocal cords and the lower part of the pharynx. The recurrent laryngeal nerve (RL) supplies the larynx below the vocal folds and the upper part of the esophagus.

NORMAL AIRWAY ANATOMY

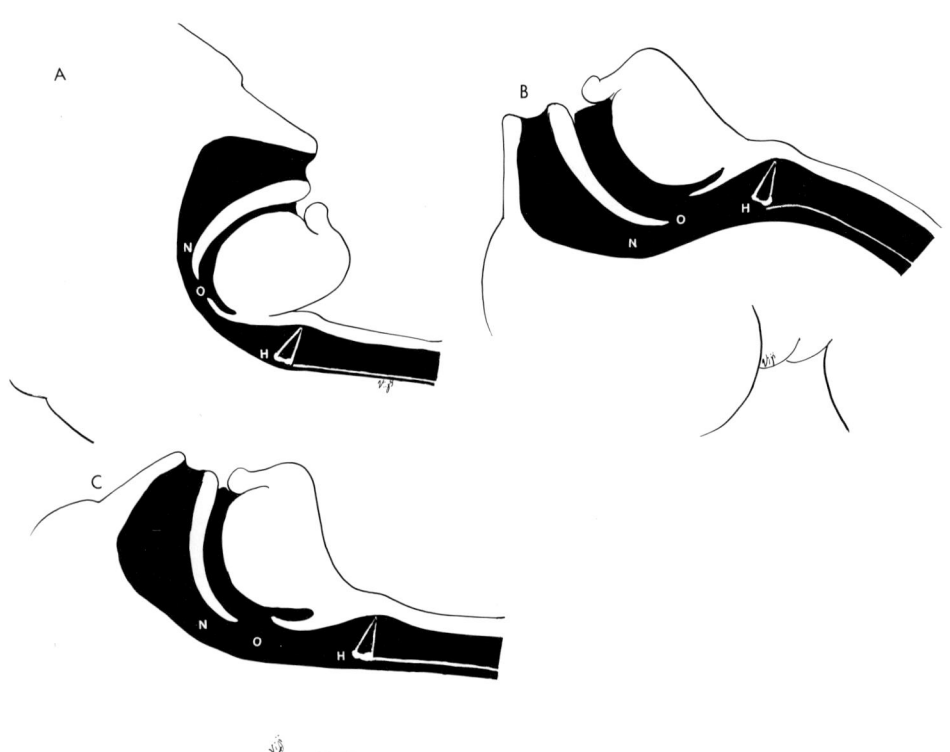

Fig 4–5.—Relationship of the nasopharynx (N), oropharynx (O), and hypopharynx (H) to the larynx with the head: **(A)** flexed; **(B)** extended; and **(C)** in the "sniffing" position.

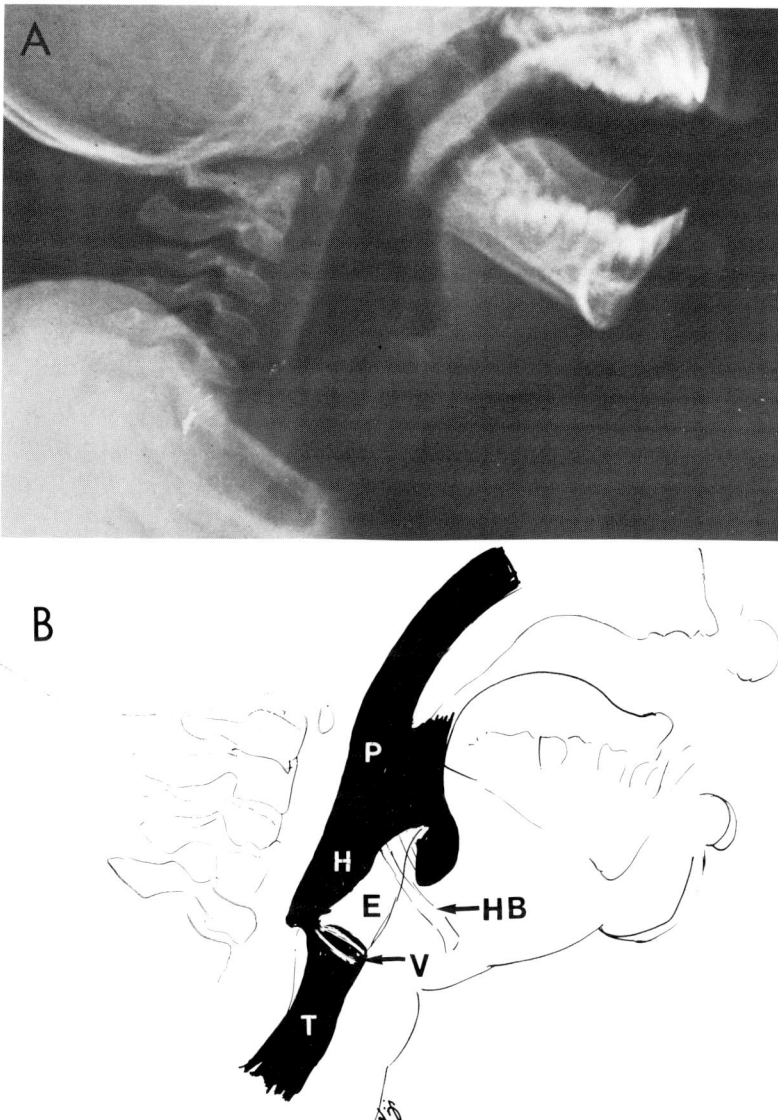

Fig 4–6.—A, lateral x-ray of the head and neck of an 18-month-old child. **B,** line drawing illustrating the position of the pharynx (P), hypopharynx (H), epiglottis (E), hyoid bone (HB), vocal folds (V), and trachea (T).

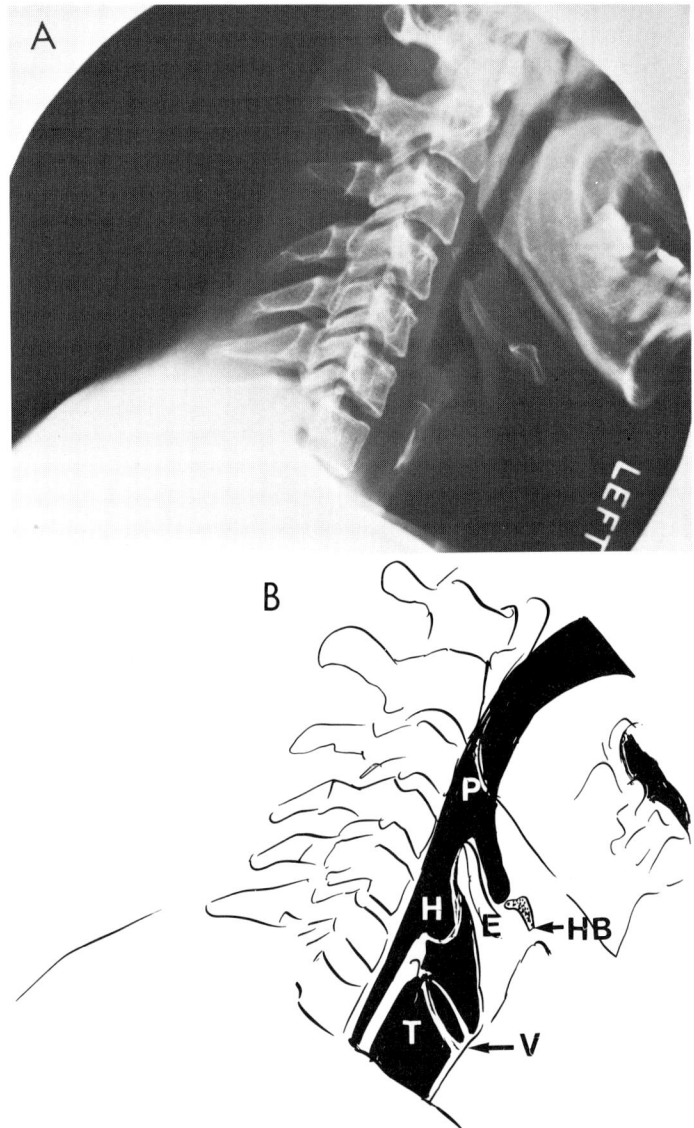

Fig 4–7.—A, lateral x-ray film of the head and neck of an adult. **B,** line drawing illustrating the position of the pharynx (P), hypopharynx (H), epiglottis (E), hyoid bone (HB), vocal folds (V), and trachea (T).

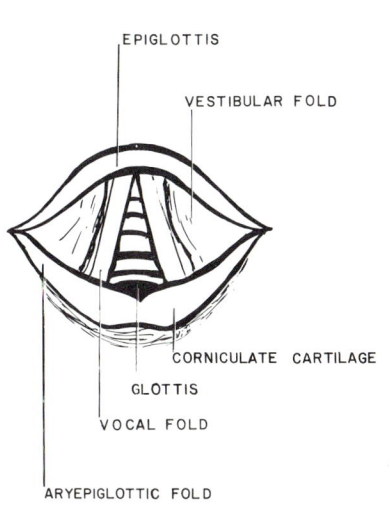 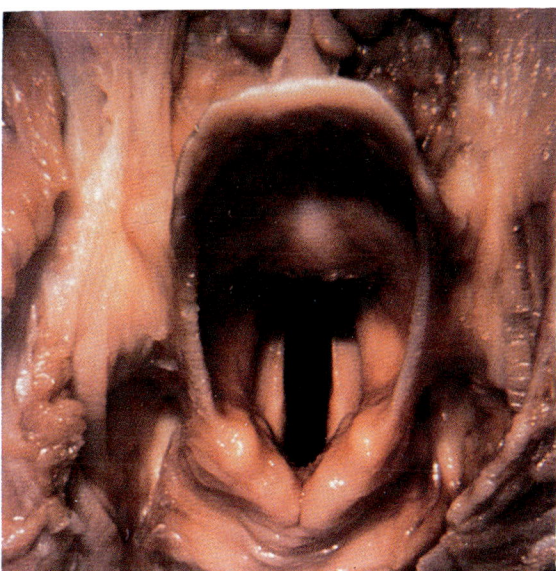

Fig 4–8.—Cadaver larynx and diagram.

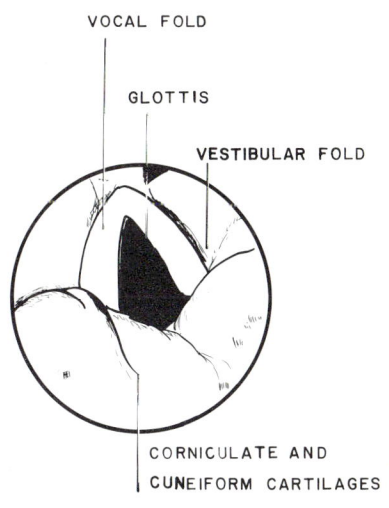 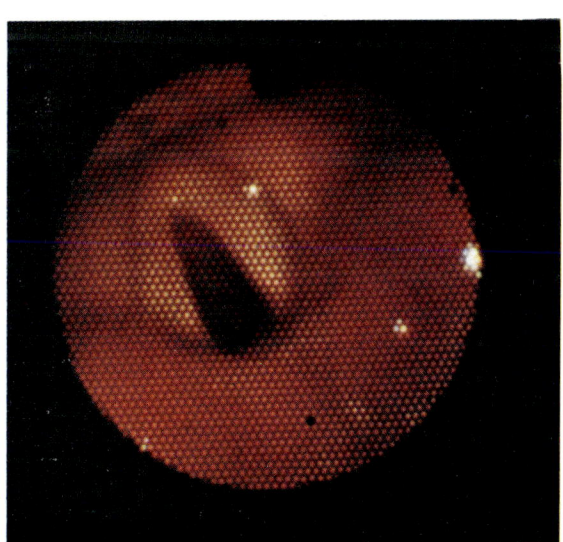

Fig 4–9.—Endoscopic view of normal larynx.

Fig 4–10.—The length of the tracheobronchial segments in adults: trachea (T), 10–11 cm; right main bronchus *(R)*, 2.5 cm; and left main bronchus *(L)*, 5.0 cm.

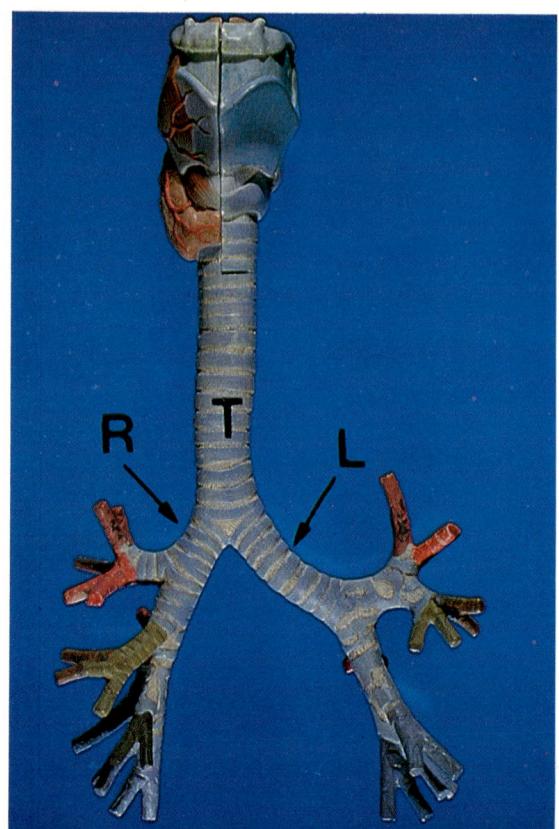

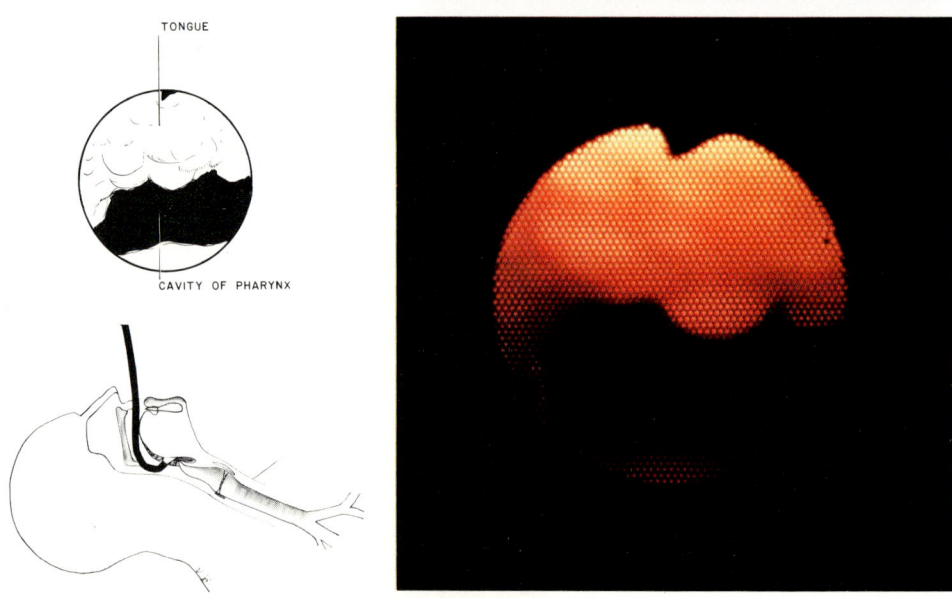

Fig 4–11.—The color of the tongue varies from white to pale pink or red. The irregular surface is produced by papillae.

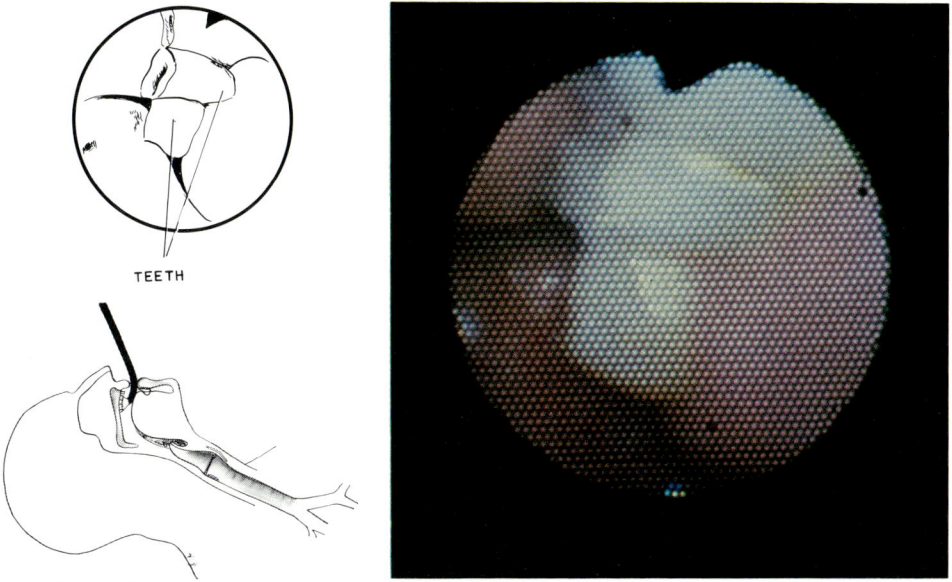

Fig 4–12.—The teeth will be visualized if the tip of the endoscope is placed superficially and not in the midline.

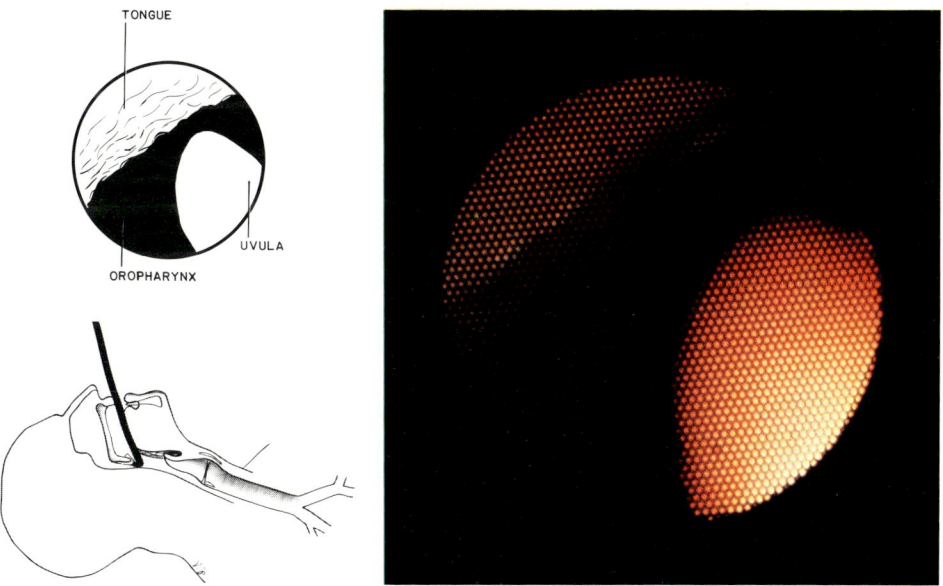

Fig 4–13.—The uvula is a smooth, oval structure in the pharynx.

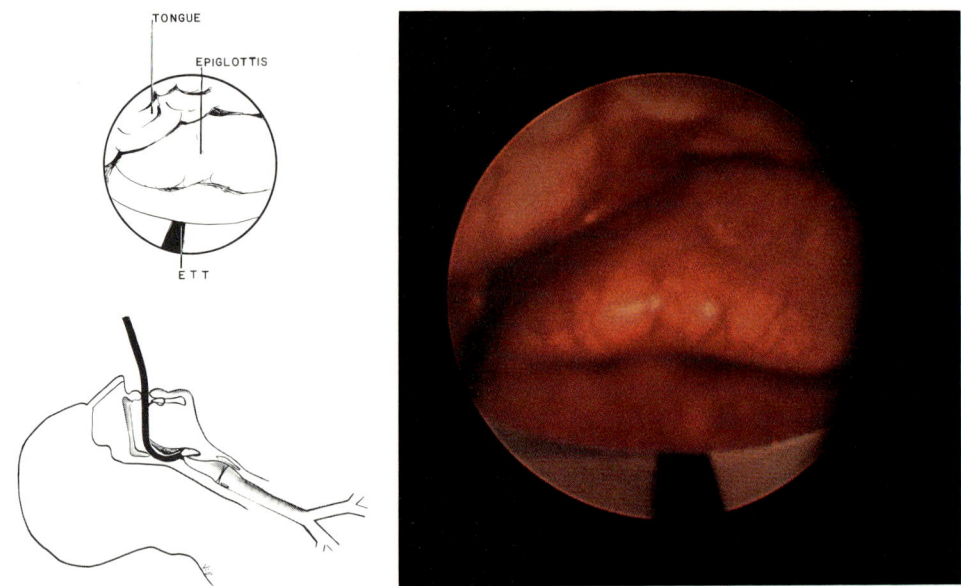

Fig 4–14.—Base of the tongue and epiglottis.

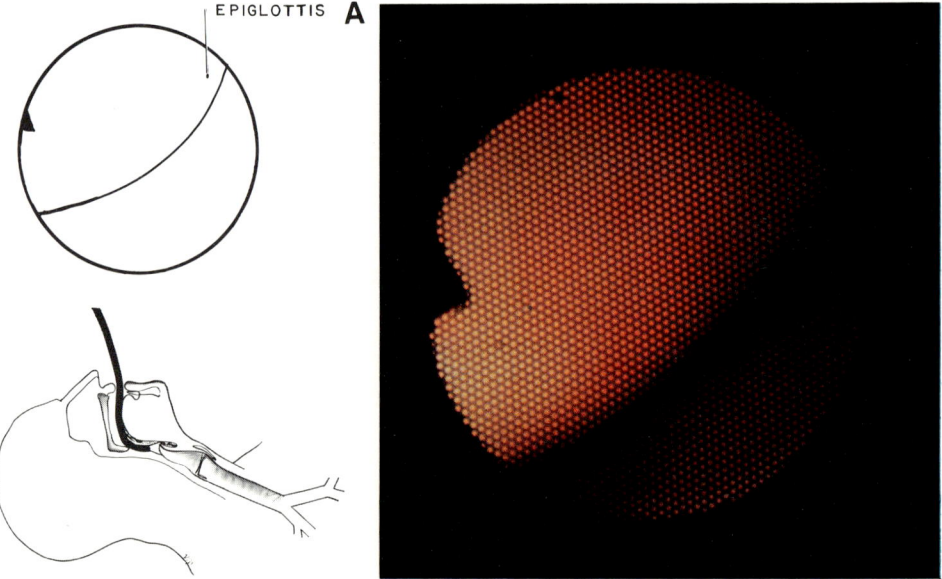

Fig 4–15.—**A,** the epiglottis, a semicircular structure with a rounded edge, moves away from the pharynx with protraction of the tongue and mandible. **B–E,** appearance of epiglottis from different angles.

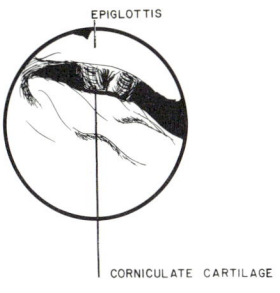

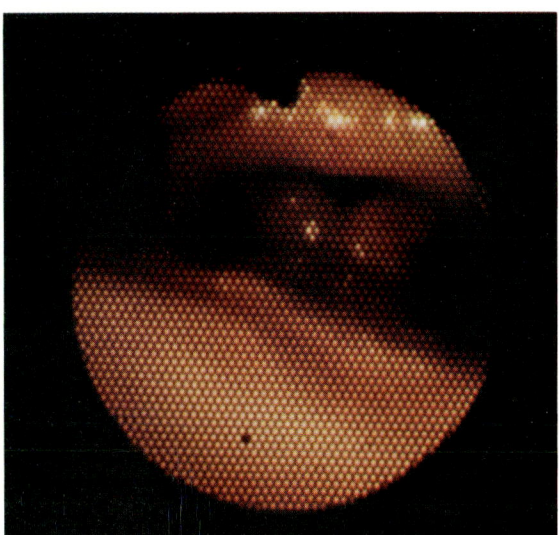

Fig 4–15 B.

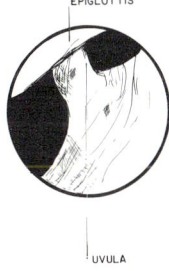

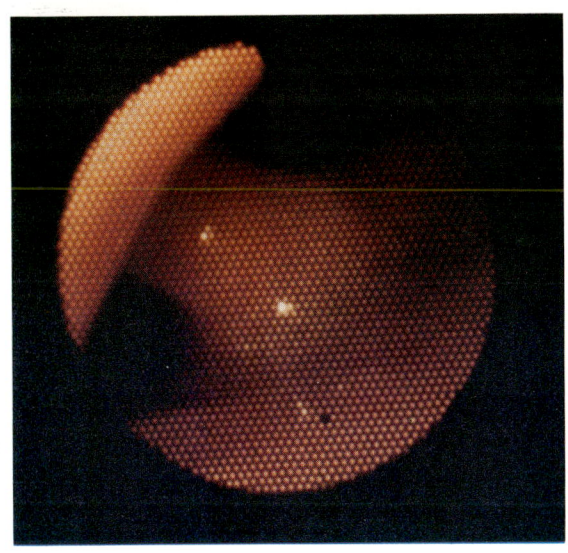

Fig 4–15 C.

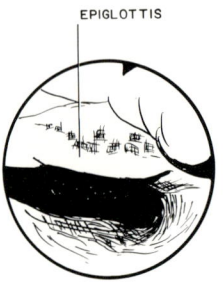
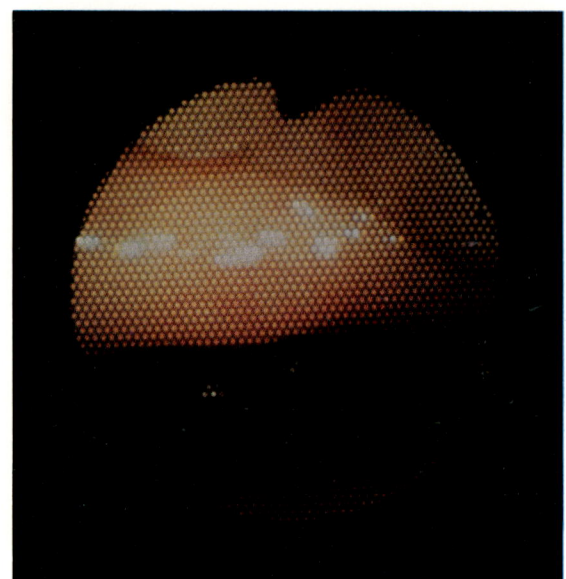

Fig 4–15 D.

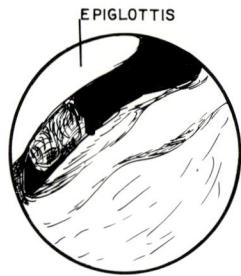
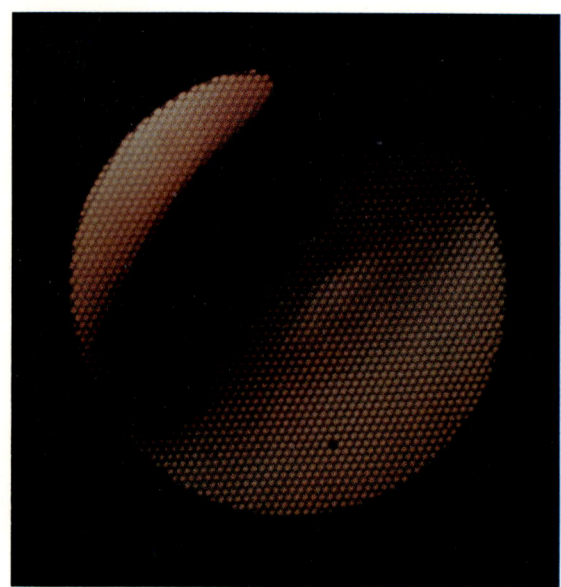

Fig 4–15 E.

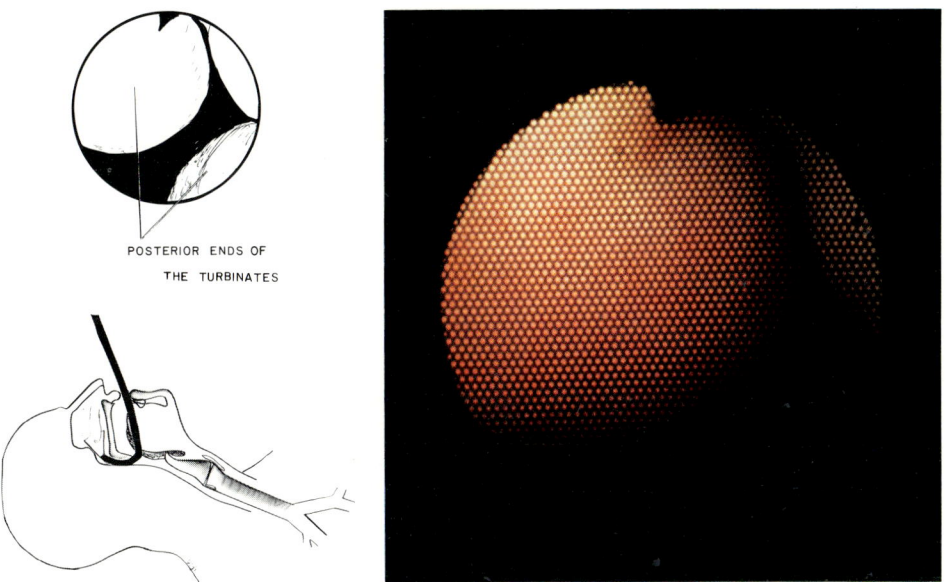

Fig 4–16.—The posterior ends of the turbinates are seen when the insertion tube is advanced too far posteriorly.

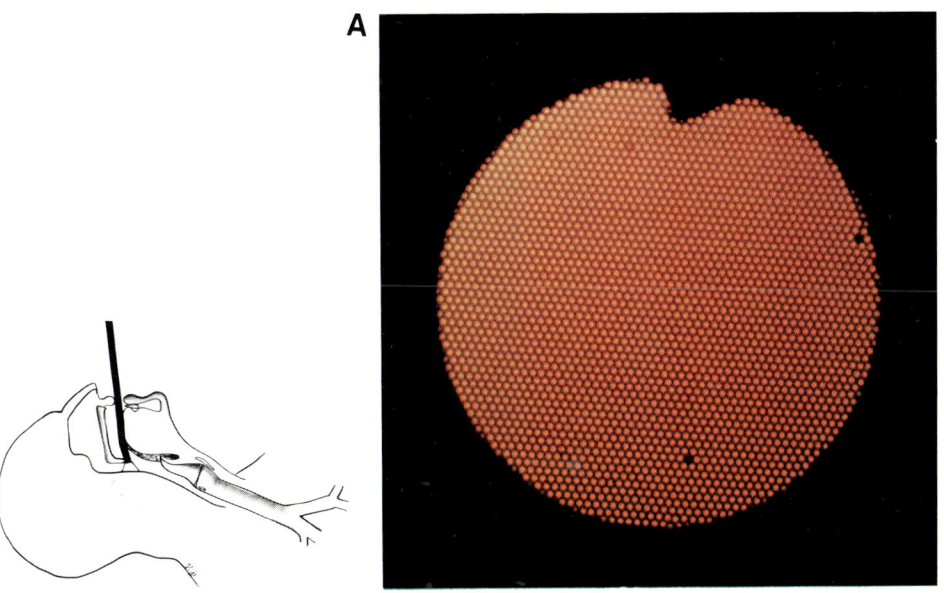

Fig 4–17.—The oropharynx is ground glass in appearance, pale pink **(A)** to red **(B),** depending on the degree of congestion. The *notch* indicates the 12 o'clock position of the lens.

55

Fig 4–17 B.

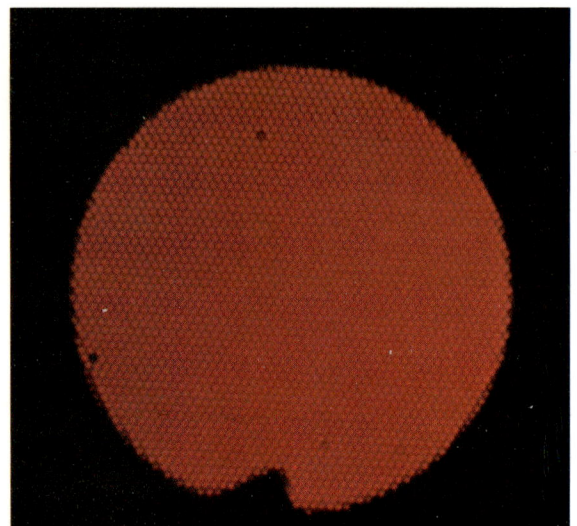

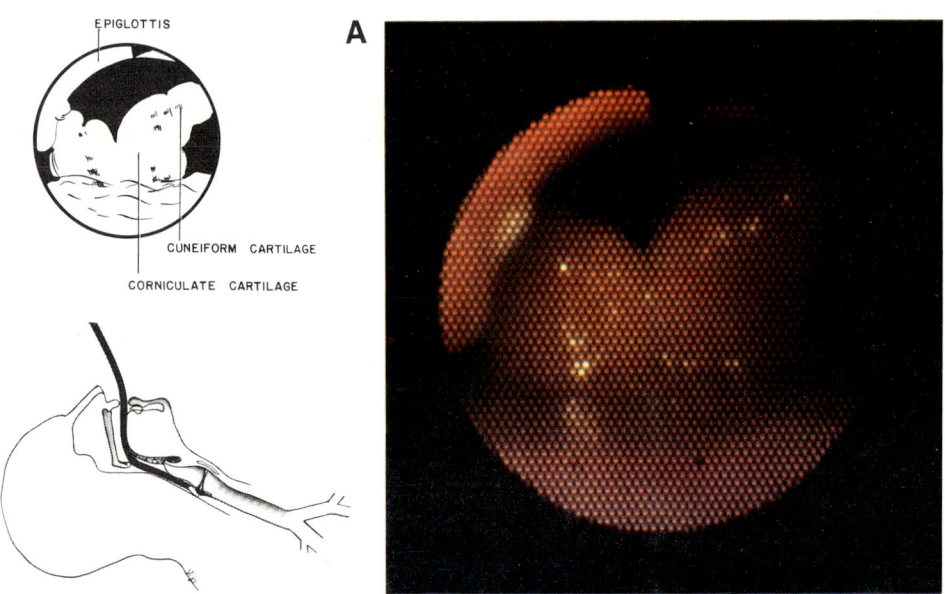

Fig 4–18.—**A–C,** the corniculate and cuneiform cartilages are often erroneously referred to as the arytenoids, which actually lie below the corniculate cartilages and are not visualized during laryngoscopy.

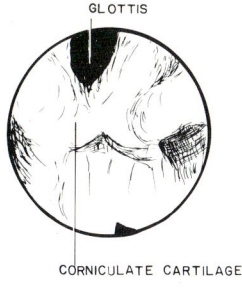

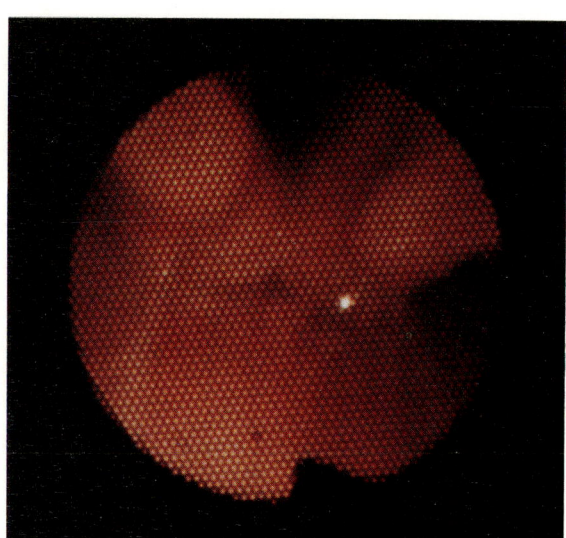

Fig 4–18 B.

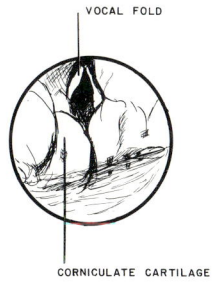

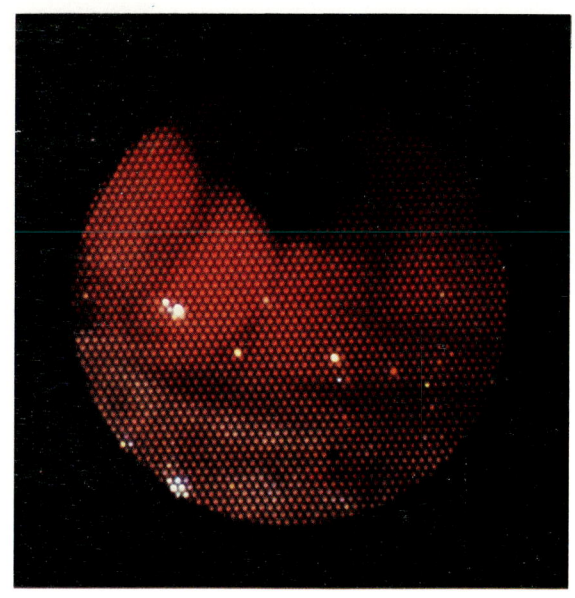

Fig 4–18 C.

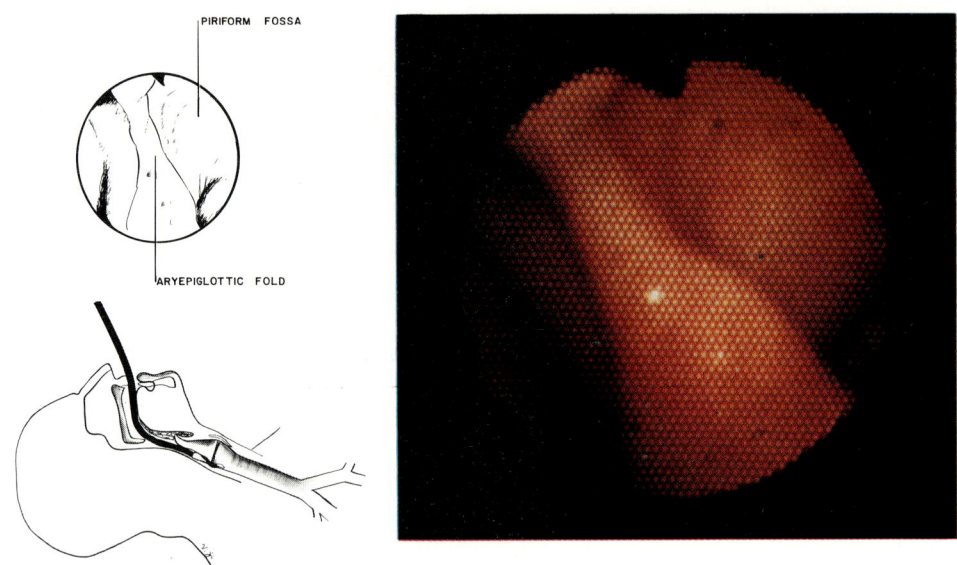

Fig 4–19.—The aryepiglottic fold runs from the corniculate cartilage to the lateral border of the epiglottis.

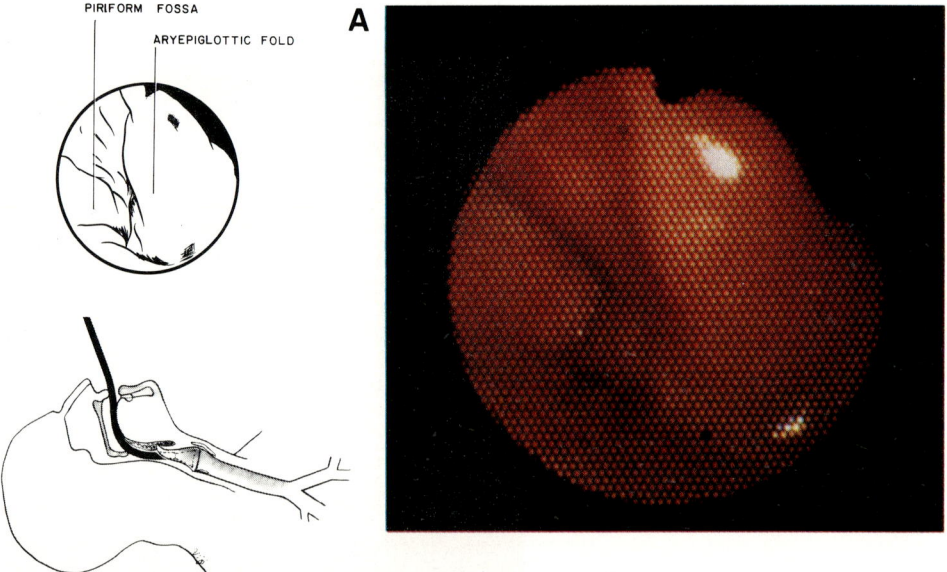

Fig 4–20.—**A–D,** the piriform fossae may be mistaken for the glottis, especially in the anesthetized patient. The tip of the endoscope can also be entrapped in this area.

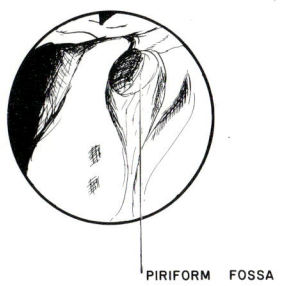
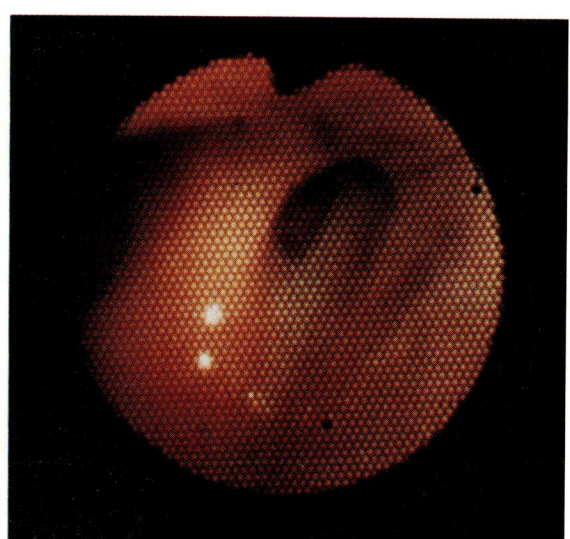

Fig 4–20 B.

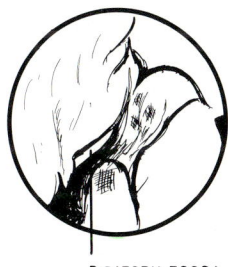
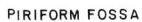
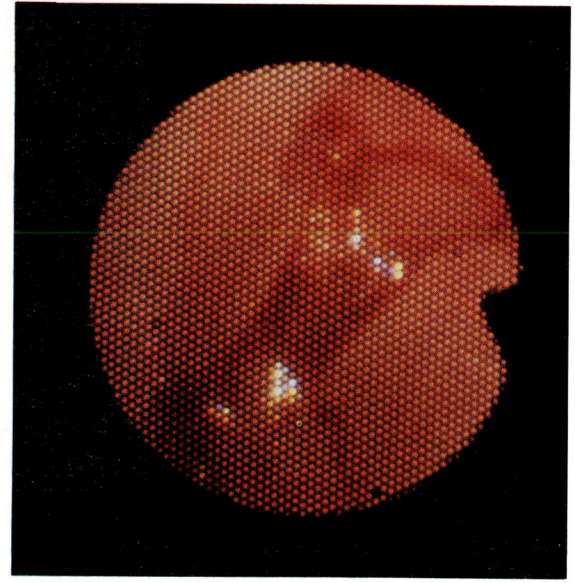

Fig 4–20 C.

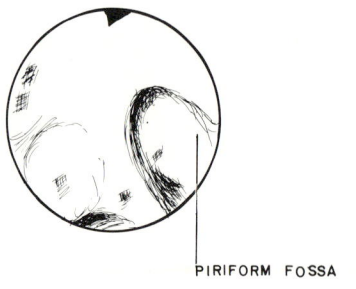
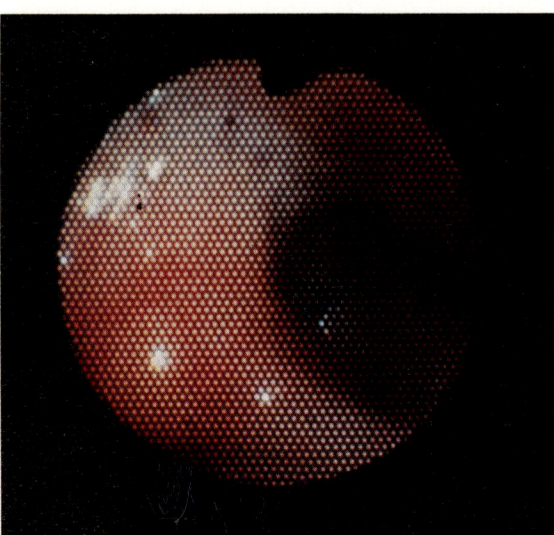

Fig 4–20 D.

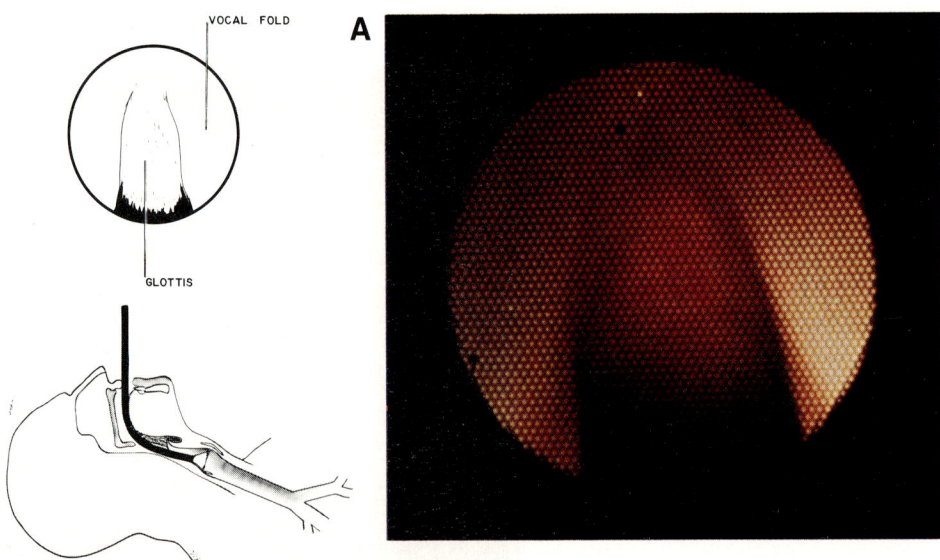

Fig 4–21.—A–C, the vocal folds are normally ivory-colored but may be pink or red if traumatized. On closer examination, they resemble tissue folds.

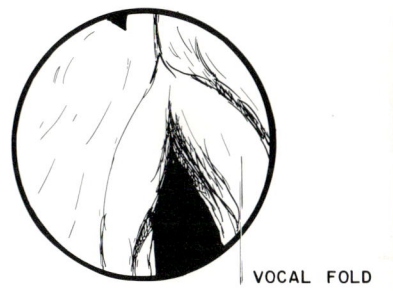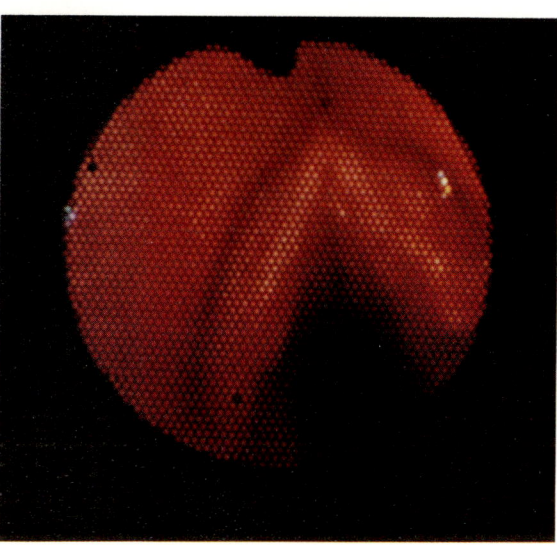

Fig 4–21 B.

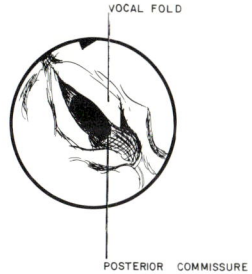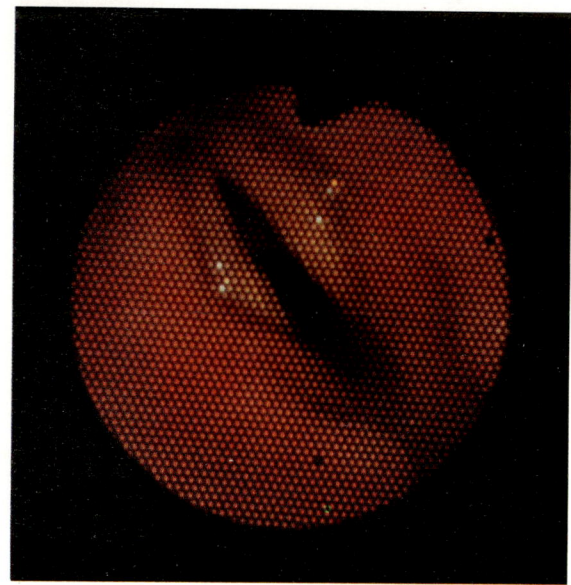

Fig 4–21 C.

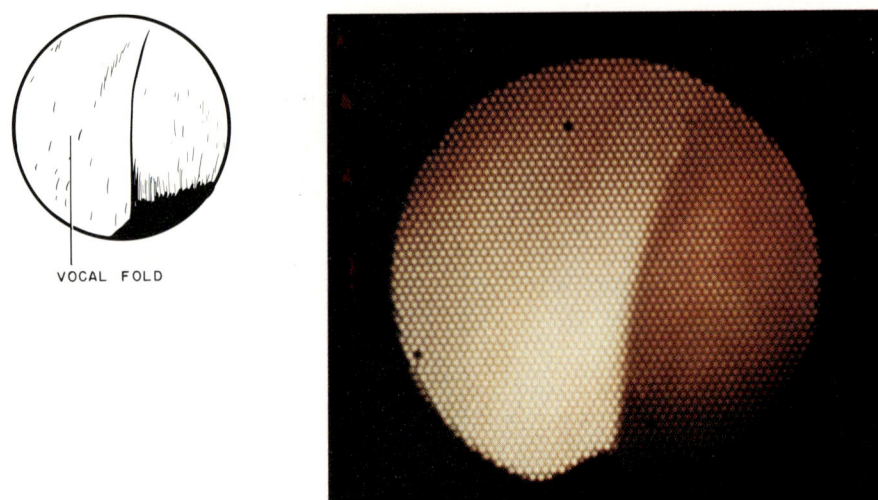

Fig 4–22.—Vocal fold.

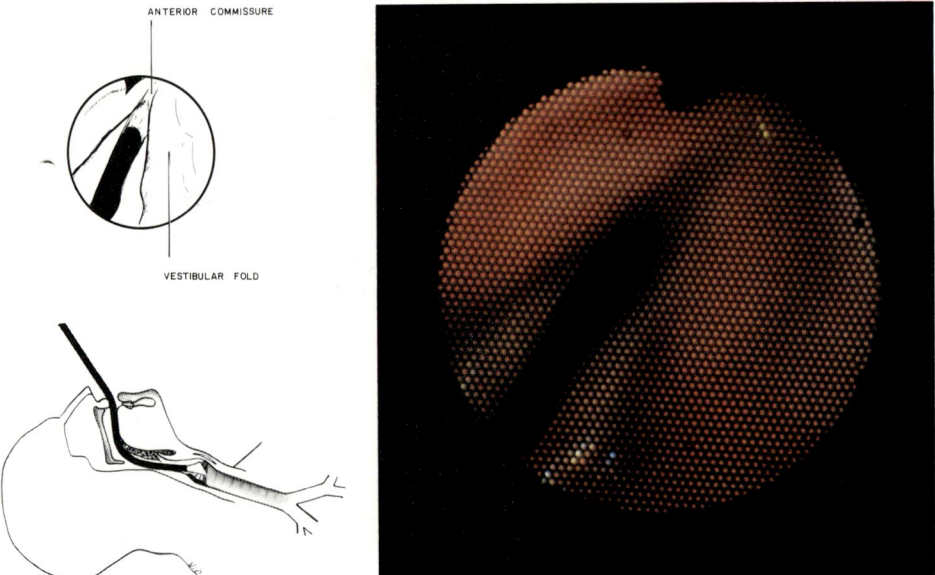

Fig 4–23.—The vestibular folds may overlie the vocal folds.

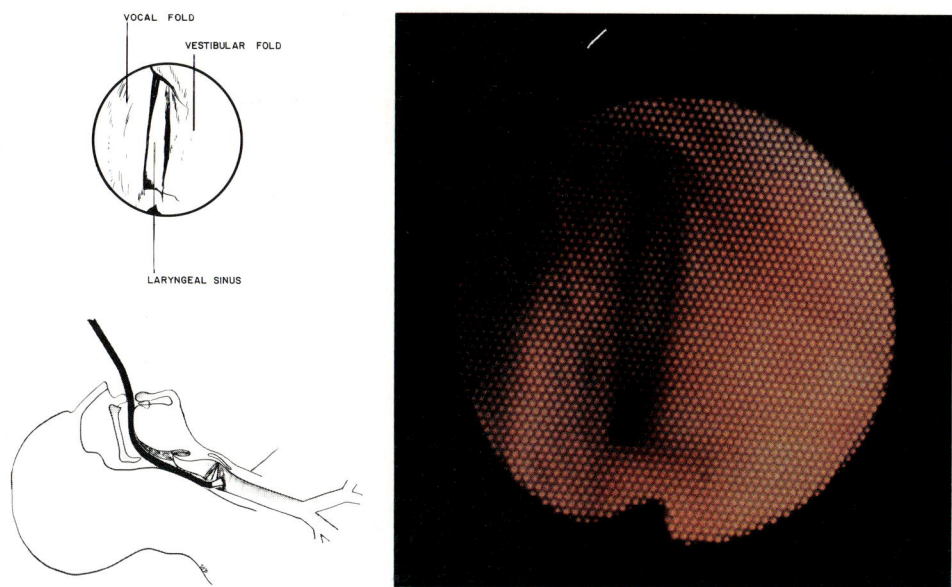

Fig 4–24.—The laryngeal sinus between the vocal folds and vestibular folds resembles a closed glottis.

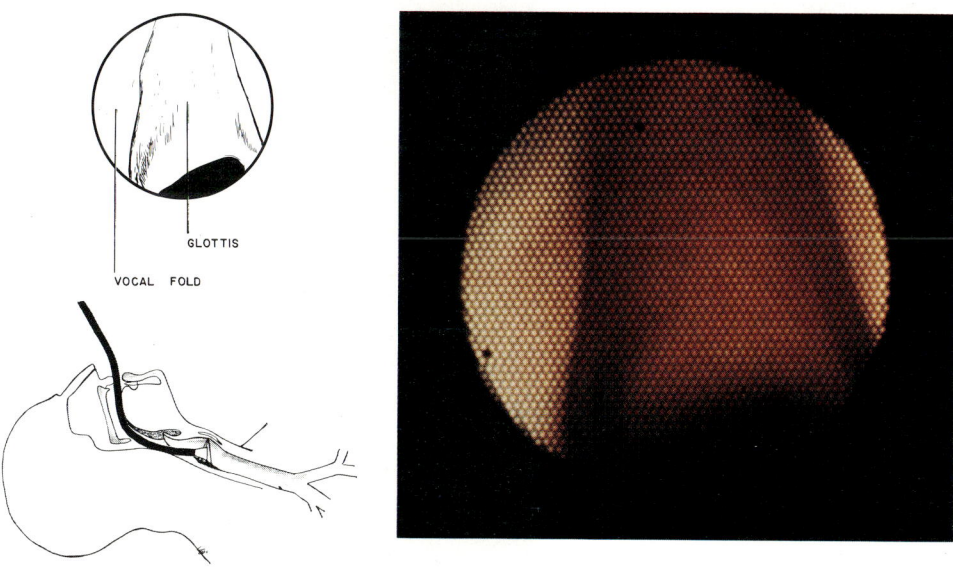

Fig 4–25.—The glottis.

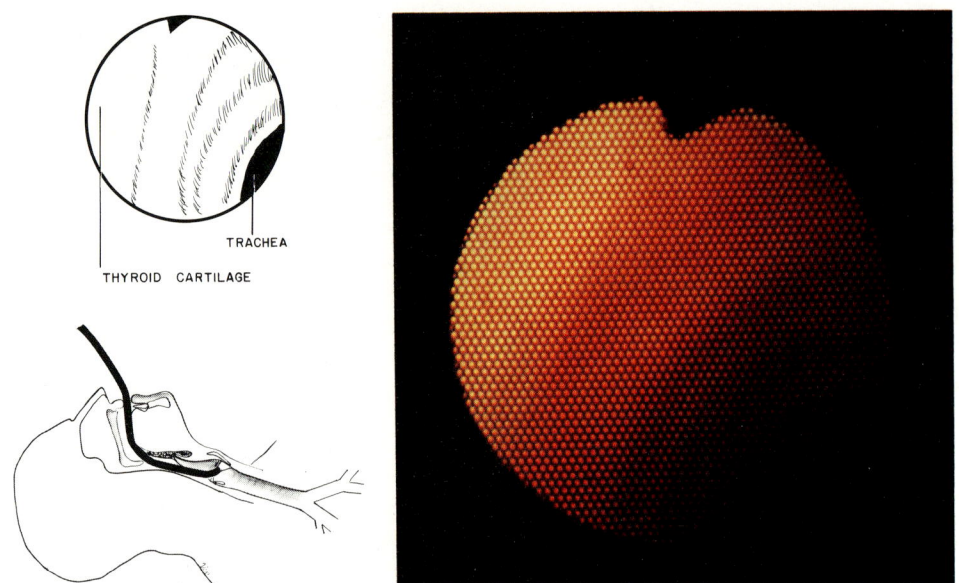

Fig 4–26.—The thyroid cartilage is viewed immediately after passing through the glottis when the endoscope tip faces anteriorly.

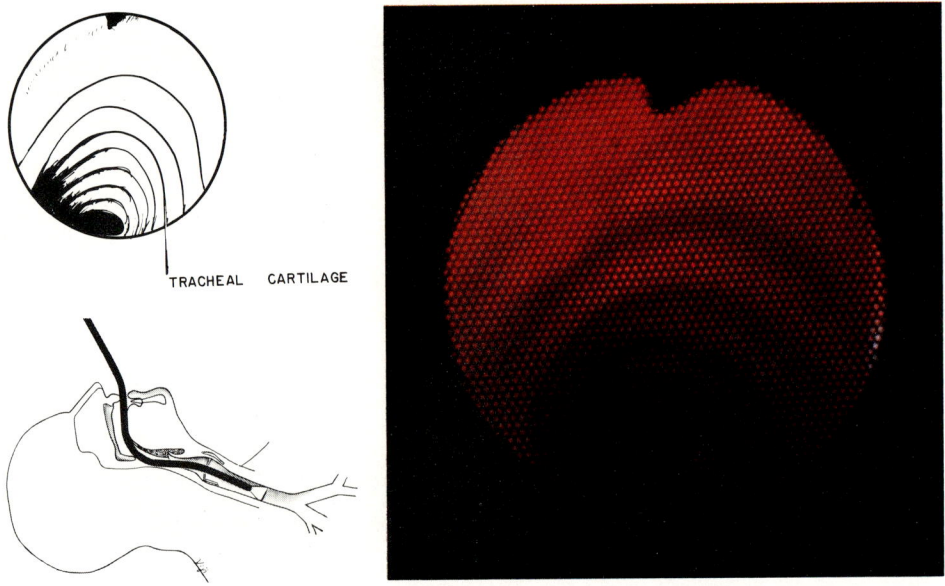

Fig 4–27.—The tracheal cartilages as visualized through the glottis.

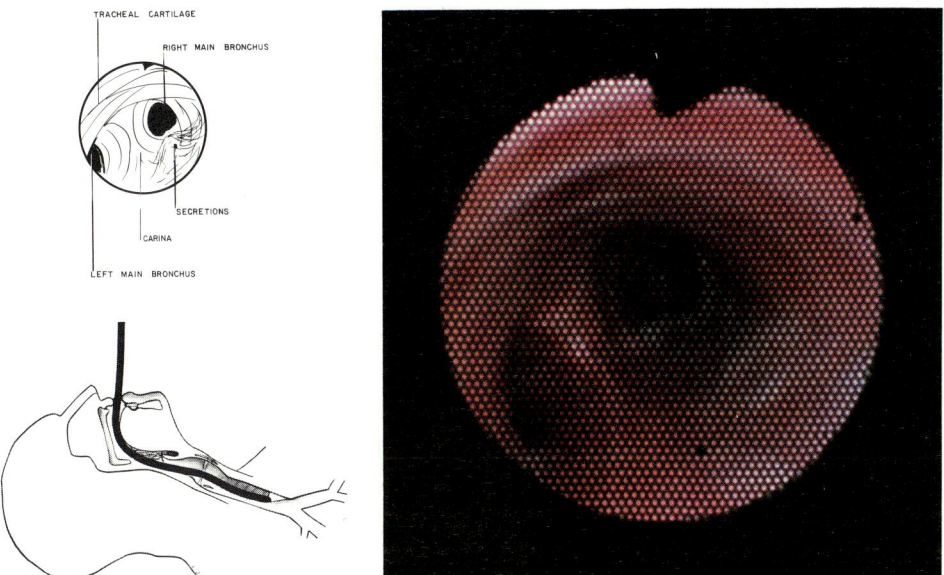

Fig 4–28.—The tracheal cartilages are covered by pale, healthy mucosa containing a fine meshwork of vessels. Intercartilaginous grooves are darker. The anterior and lateral walls of the trachea are identified by the presence of cartilaginous rings.

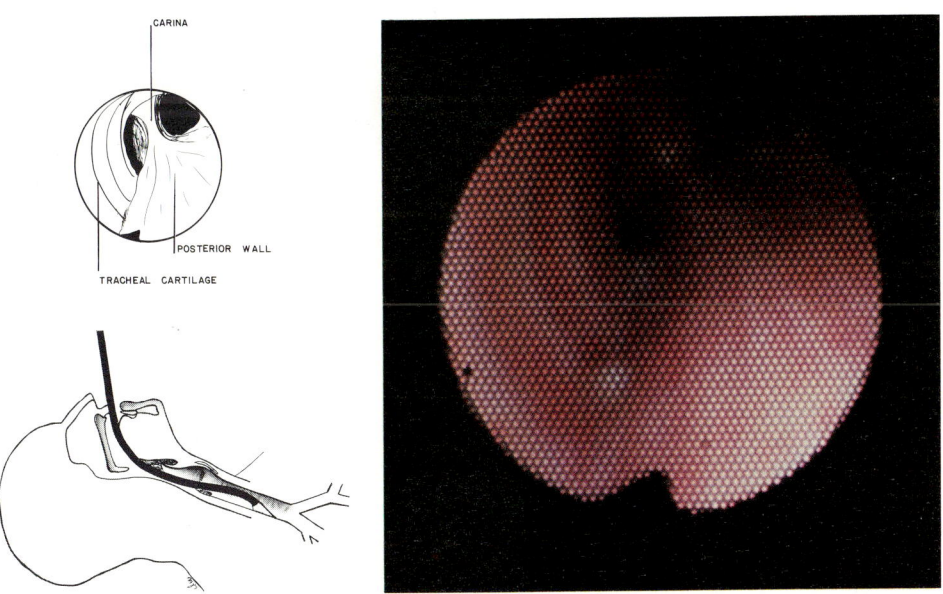

Fig 4–29.—The posterior wall of the trachea is membranous, noncartilaginous, and bulges into the lumen during expiration.

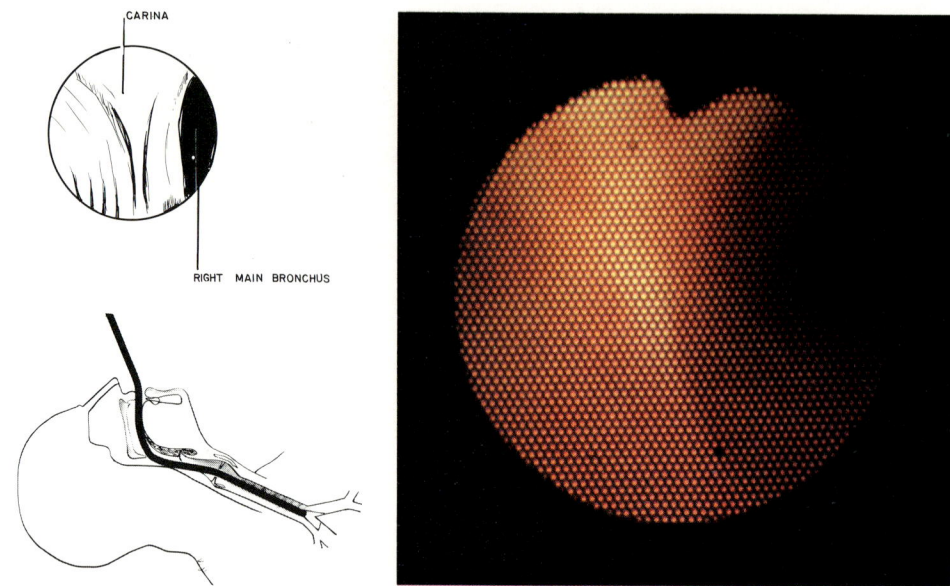

Fig 4–30.—The normal carina has a sharp edge. The mucosa appears bright or pale red, depending on the amount of light reflected.

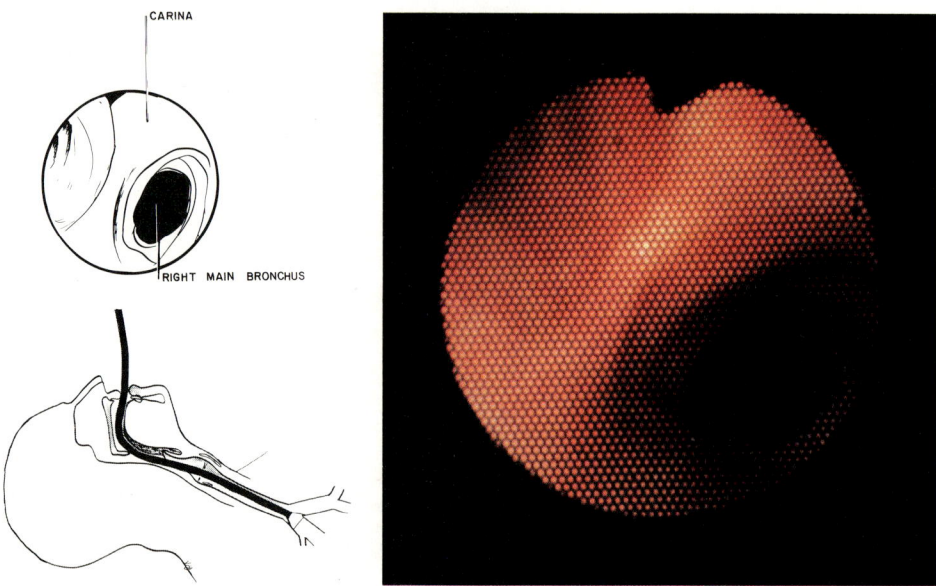

Fig 4–31.—The right main bronchus is wider, shorter, and more vertical than the left.

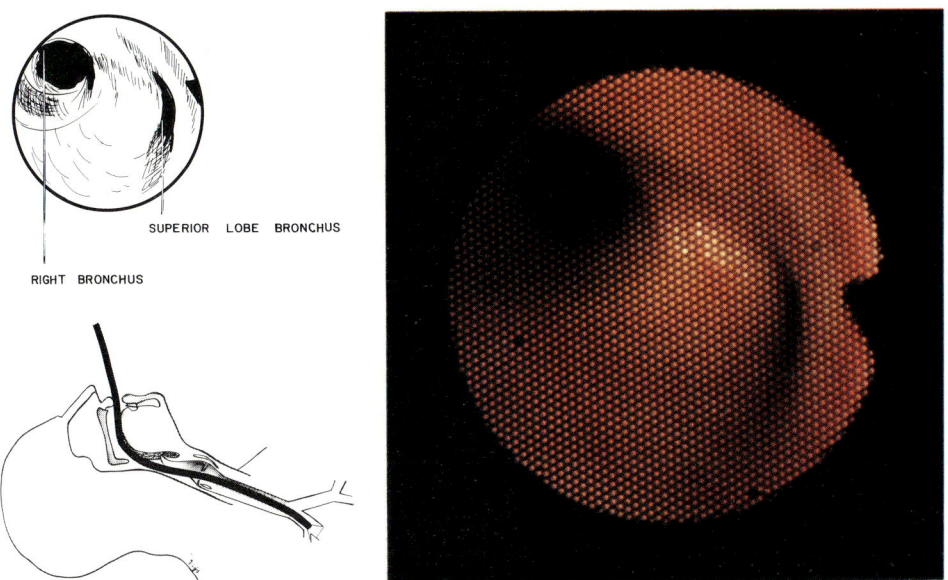

Fig 4–32.—The right superior lobe bronchus arises from the lateral aspect of the right main bronchus.

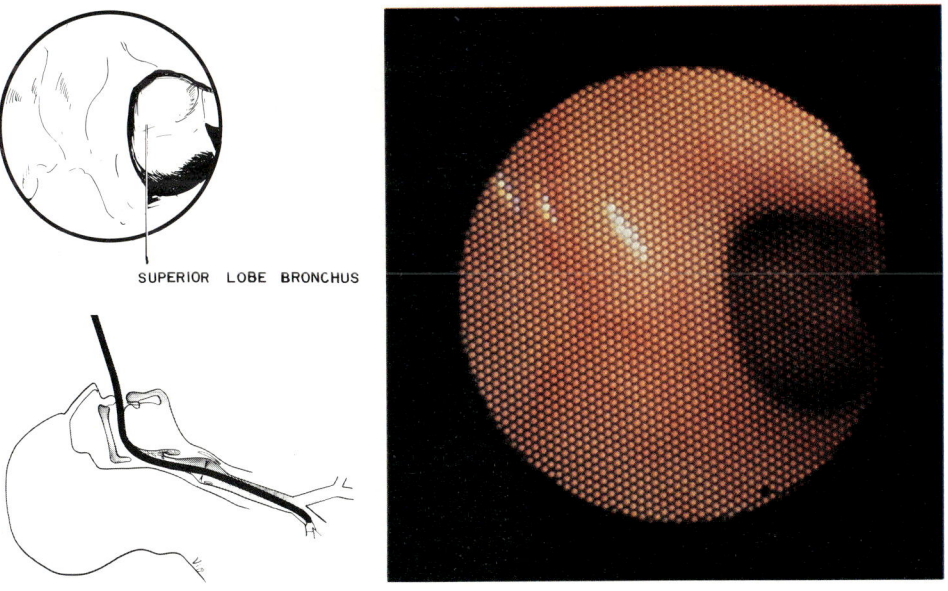

Fig 4–33.—The right superior lobe bronchus.

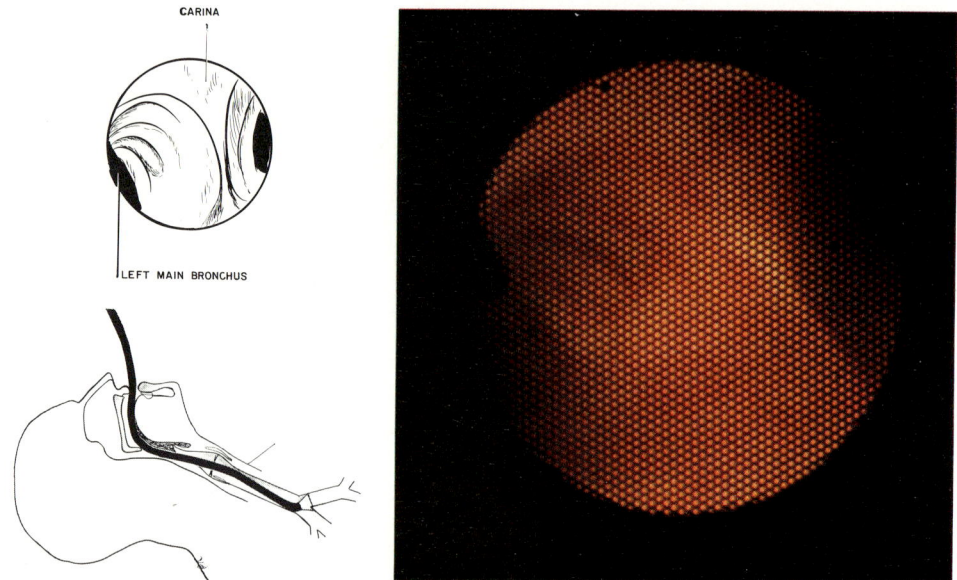

Fig 4–34.—The lumen of the left main bronchus is not seen until the endoscope is advanced farther, since it is more acutely placed than the right.

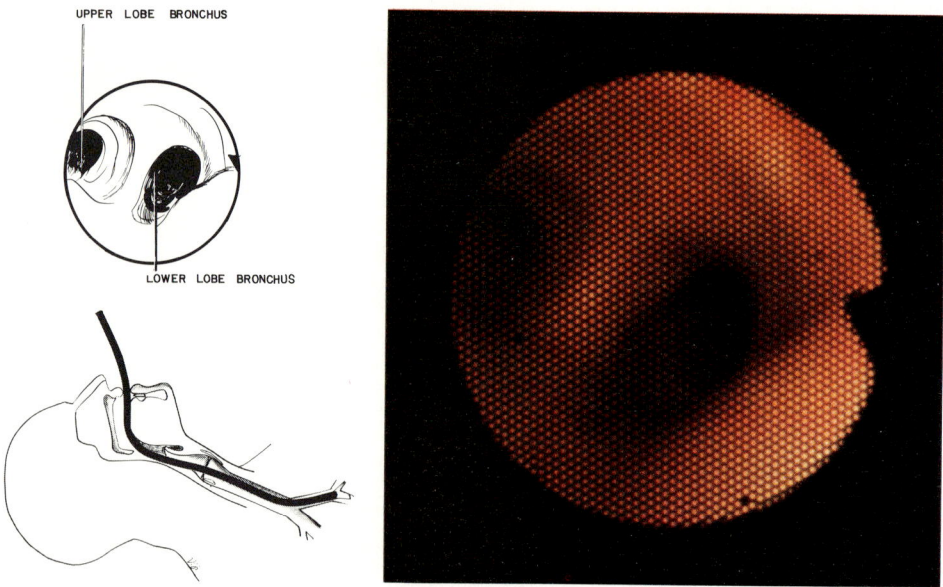

Fig 4–35.—Segments of the left main bronchus.

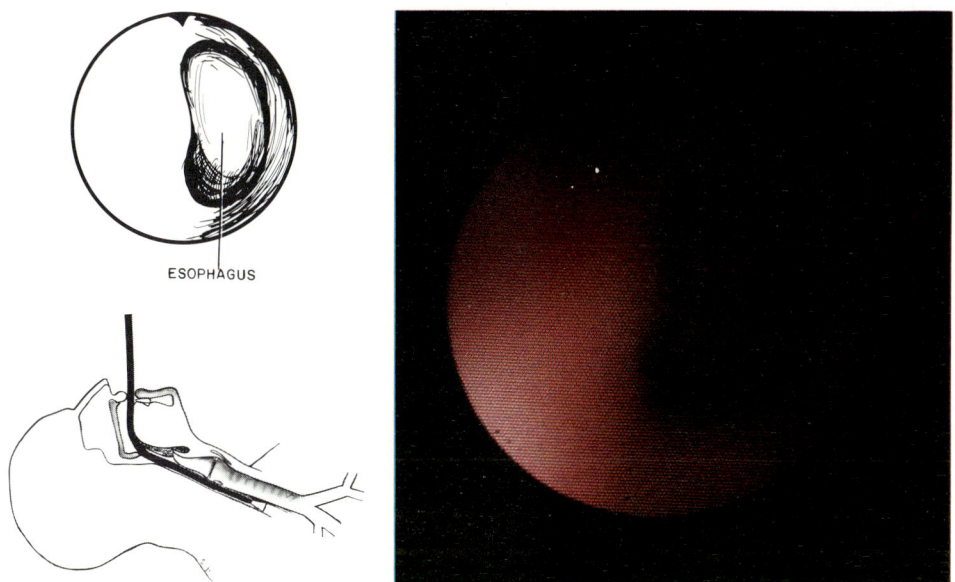

Fig 4–36.—The esophagus is pink or red, and the wall collapses over the endoscope.

THE AIRWAY OF THE INFANT

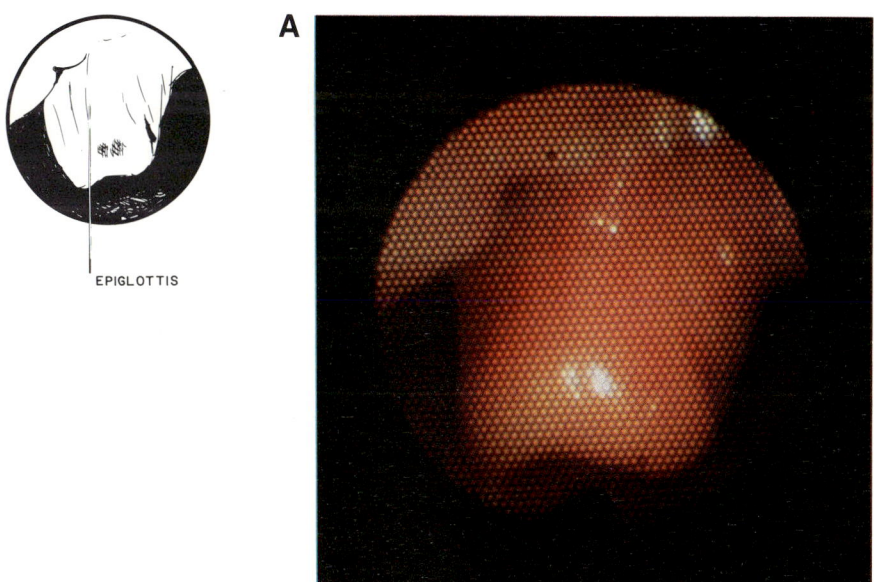

Fig 4–37.—**A–C,** the epiglottis is narrow, and the angle between the glottis and epiglottis is more acute than in the adult.

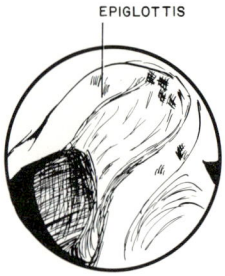

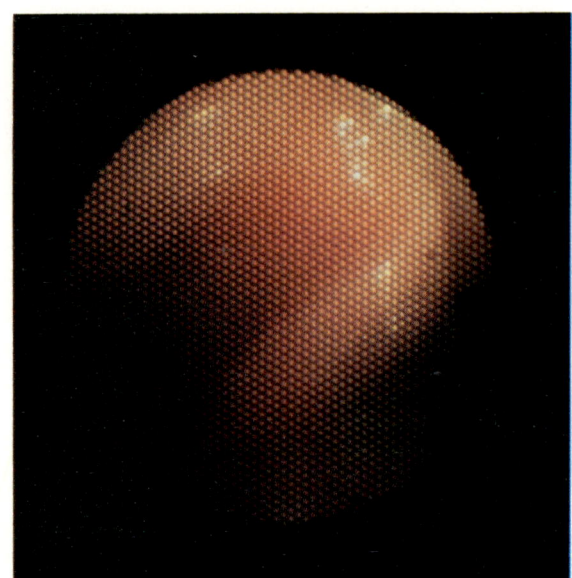

Fig 4–37 B.

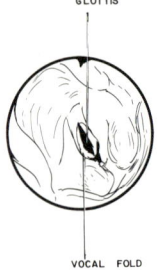

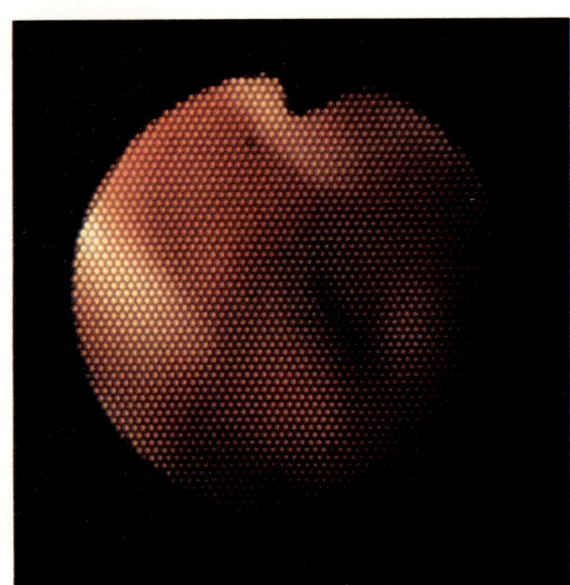

Fig 4–37 C.

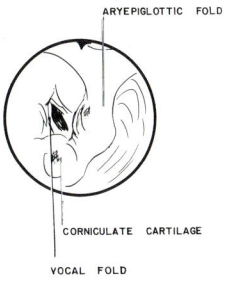
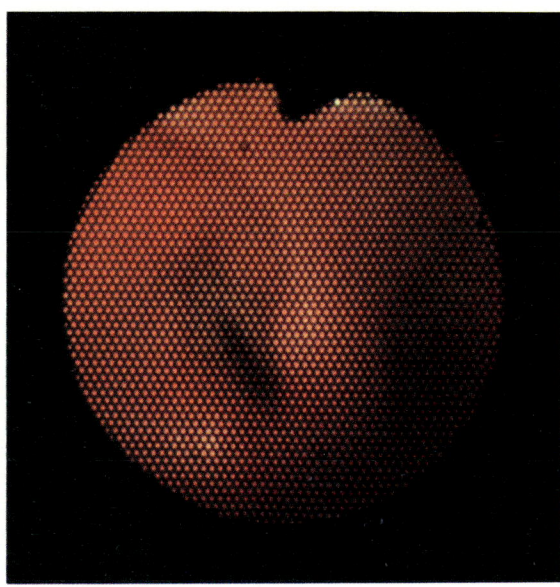

Fig 4–38.—The aryepiglottic folds are prominent.

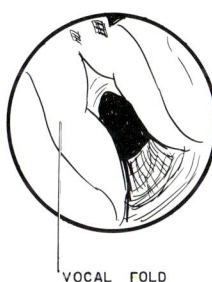
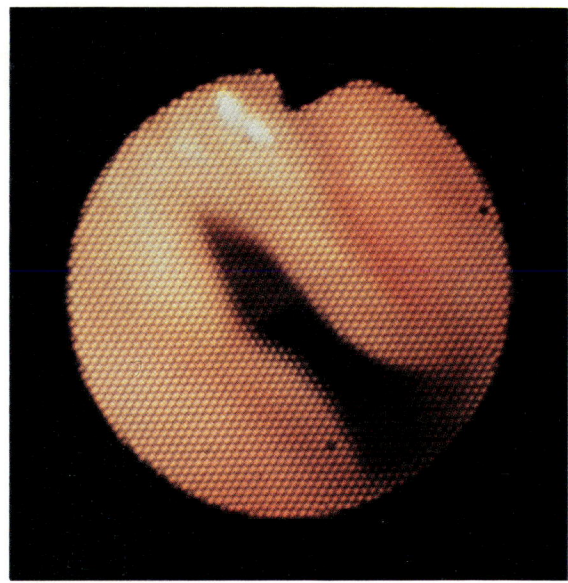

Fig 4–39.—The vocal folds.

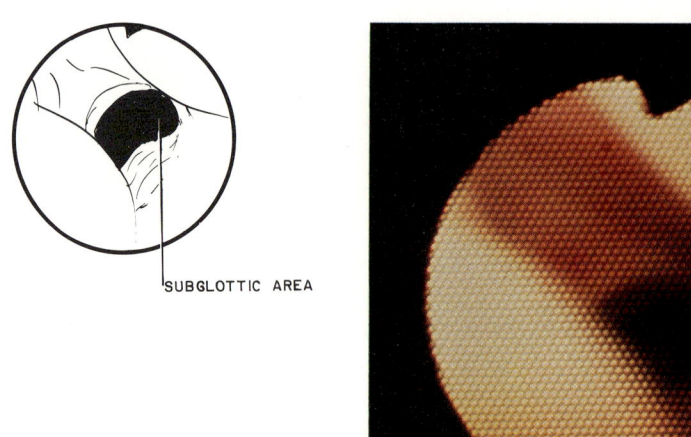

Fig 4–40.—The subglottic area.

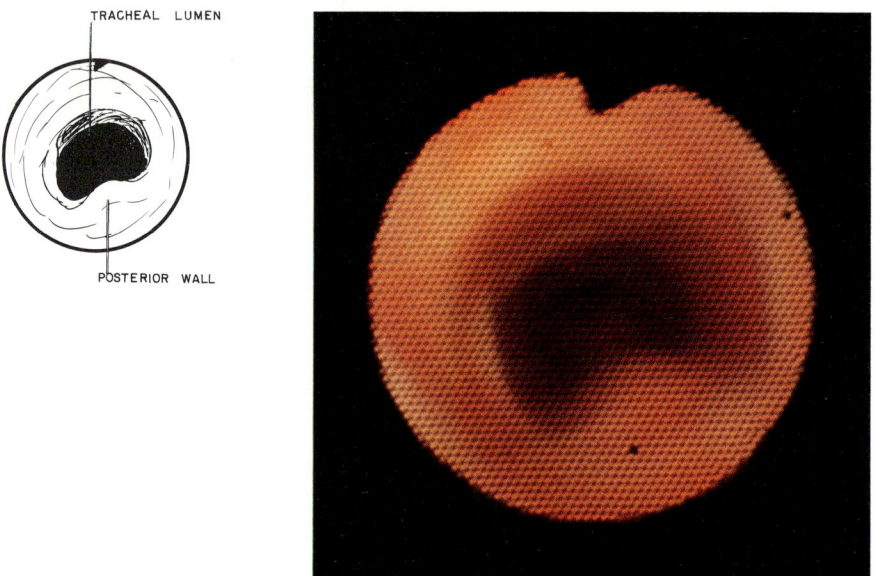

Fig 4–41.—The posterior wall of the trachea bulges into the lumen during expiration.

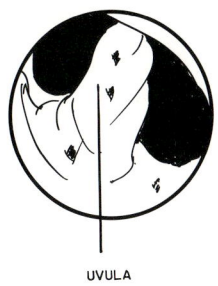
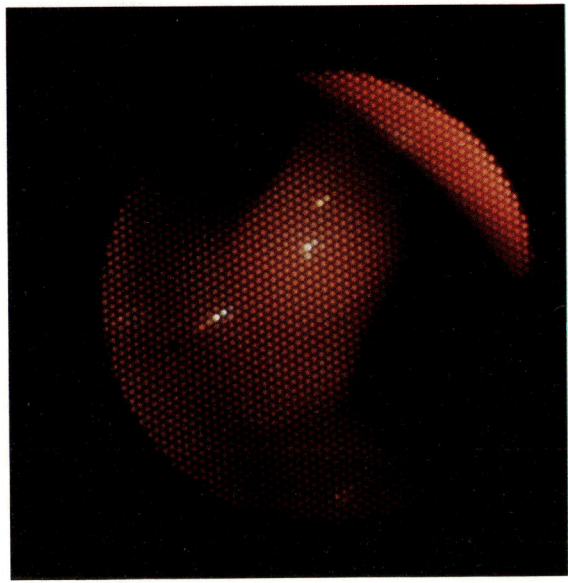

Fig 4–42.—The uvula is relatively long and narrow.

5 / Techniques of Endotracheal Intubation

THE KEYS TO SUCCESSFUL fiberoptic laryngoscopy are preparation, patience, and practice. Frequently, the technique is undertaken after multiple unsuccessful attempts at intubation have resulted in tissue trauma, edema, and bleeding. In such circumstances anatomical landmarks are obscured and there is little chance of success. A vicious cycle ensues: the endoscopist is frustrated, endotracheal intubation is impossible, and more frustration develops. If general anesthesia is administered, the patient either is inadequately anesthetized or receives excessive doses of IV agents. If topical anesthesia is used, the patient is exhausted, uncooperative, restless, and miserable. The same adjectives usually apply to the surgeon and operating room personnel.

BECOMING FAMILIAR WITH THE INSTRUMENT

Although the experienced endoscopist makes the procedure appear simple, fiberoptic laryngoscopy is a technique that must be mastered. Initial practice should be gained on an intubation mannequin—not on patients. The endoscopist is afforded the opportunity to practice at leisure on an immobile model that does not fog the lens, is free of secretions and blood, and requires no anesthesia. Time is not a consideration because the "patient" is not subject to hypoxia, cooperation is not necessary, and there is no impatient surgeon waiting. The anatomy is normal and usually larger than life-size. When practicing with the mannequin, the anesthesiologist must concentrate on developing a step-by-step routine. After gaining facility with the instrument, he should first use it in normal patients when endotracheal intubation is indicated. Only after successfully intubating several patients who have normal airway anatomy should the anesthesiologist attempt to use the instrument when difficulty with intubation is anticipated.

THE TECHNIQUE

The first step must always be a check of the working elements of the endoscope and the light source prior to use. While not necessary when one is practicing on a mannequin, application of an antifog agent to the lens is mandatory when the instrument is used in patients. The lens should be focused prior to use, not after the instrument is inserted. The sheath of the insertion tube is thoroughly lubricated with a water-soluble jelly, beginning at the distal end and moving proximally to avoid the lens. Products containing oil or petroleum jelly are contraindicated.

The endotracheal tube (ETT) is selected relative to the type of endoscope and patient's size. The connector is removed and the tube is cut to the appropriate length since longer tubes are much more difficult to manipulate. Visibility is enhanced if a constant flow of oxygen (2–3 L/minute) is maintained through the operating channel. In addition to providing a higher inspired oxygen concentration, the oxygen forces mucus, blood, and secretions away from the lens of the endoscope. Incorporating a three-way stopcock in the suction tube allows alternating suction and oxygen flow.

An assistant is desirable when the procedure is performed with topical anesthesia and mandatory if general anesthesia is administered. The ETT is threaded over the well-lubricated insertion tube. The control section is held in one hand, with the thumb positioned on the angle control and the index finger on the suction port. The insertion tube is held straight with the other hand, and the angle knob is manipulated to insure that the end of the tube moves up and down, not sideways. In the adult patient the insertion tube is advanced 8–10 cm into the pharynx. It is imperative that the tube remain in the midline. This is most easily achieved by using an endoscopic airway that has a central groove to maintain the midline position of the insertion tube as it is advanced. At this time the anesthesiologist looks into the endoscope and identifies the structures visualized. If the tube is in the midline and has been advanced the proper distance, the vocal cords will come into view as the tip of the scope is flexed upward. A local anesthetic agent can be instilled through the suction port directly onto the vocal cords if laryngeal anesthesia is inadequate. Slight rotation of the insertion tube may be required to bring the tip into the midline. The endoscope is then advanced through the vocal cords. The first view after the vocal cords will not be the tracheal cartilages, but the thyroid cartilage. The tip of the endoscope is straightened or returned to the neutral position and advanced until the tracheal cartilages, and finally the carina, are seen. The endoscope is held firmly just above the carina, the ETT is threaded into the trachea, and the endoscope removed. The instrument should be cleaned immediately after use.

REASONS FOR FAILURE

The image will be blurred or hazy if there is insufficient light or if the instrument is not focused. Secretions and blood can obscure the lens, and it will become fogged after several minutes of use. The solutions to the first problems are obvious. If suctioning or flowing oxygen through the channel does not improve vision, the instrument must be withdrawn, cleaned, and defogged. Broken fibers produce blind spots or dark areas. When many fibers are damaged, the fiberoptic bundle must be replaced because individual fibers cannot be repaired.

The most frequent complaint of the beginning endoscopist is "everything looks red or pink." The first reaction is to withdraw the insertion tube, presuming that the esophagus was intubated. If the endoscope advances easily greater than 10 or 12 cm beyond the pharynx and no definable structures are evident, it can be assumed that the esophagus has been entered. However, the most likely explanation is that the insertion tube is not in the midline, and the tip is facing the piriform or tonsillar fossae or the oropharynx. The endoscope should be withdrawn and reinserted to a depth of 8–10 cm. It may be necessary to remove the instrument and defog it before proceeding.

PLANNING THE ANESTHETIC

Even in expert hands, fiberoptic laryngoscopy requires more time than conventional laryngoscopy. The patient, surgeon, and operating room personnel must understand the indications for the procedure and the additional time requirement. It is imperative that the anesthetic technique be planned in advance, allowing sufficient time for induction of general anesthesia or for topical anesthesia and IV sedation to become effective.

The anesthetic technique must be chosen on the basis of the patient's anatomy, the indications for endotracheal intubation, and the experience of the endoscopist. Whenever appropriate instrumentation and experienced personnel are available, fiberoptic endoscopy can be employed equally well in pediatric patients.

REGIONAL AND TOPICAL ANESTHESIA

Topical anesthesia and transtracheal and internal laryngeal nerve blocks may be used in patients scheduled for *elective* surgery who have normal airway anatomy or in whom difficulty with airway management is anticipated. Local anesthesia may be supplemented with IV sedation. It must be remembered that local anesthetic agents and sedatives are not immediately effective and laryngoscopy should not be attempted until adequate effects are achieved.

GENERAL ANESTHESIA

Most patients prefer general anesthesia for endotracheal intubation. Only small doses of fixed agents, such as thiopental and narcotics, are used because spontaneous ventilation must be maintained. A potent inhalation agent is the primary anesthetic. Omission of nitrous oxide allows a greater margin of safety but its use is acceptable in many patients. No muscle relaxant is administered until correct placement of the ETT has been ascertained by auscultation of the chest.

Use of an endoscopic mask permits uninterrupted anesthesia and ventilation during the procedure. It is especially advantageous when an experienced endoscopist is teaching the technique because ventilation is continued and speed is not crucial. As an alternative, adequate anesthesia and ventilation can be maintained in most patients with a binasal airway to which the anesthetic circuit is attached.

OROTRACHEAL VS. NASOTRACHEAL INTUBATION

A larger ETT can be used and the potential for tissue trauma and bleeding is lower with an orotracheal tube. However, it may be difficult to thread the endotracheal tube once the endoscope is within the trachea because of the acute angle formed by the oropharynx and trachea. Retraction of the tongue and protrusion of the mandible are usually effective in overcoming this problem. If the bevel of the tube is caught at the level of the epiglottis or aryepiglottic folds, slight rotation of the ETT combined with forward displacement of the tongue will usually disengage the tube and allow it to slide through the vocal cords. The largest endoscope that will fit easily into the endotracheal tube should be used because it is more difficult to thread a large ETT over a small, flexible endoscope.

Nasotracheal intubation is contraindicated in the patient with clotting abnormalities. Although topical vasoconstrictors such as cocaine or phenylephrine decrease bleeding, visibility may be hampered by the presence of blood and secretions. It is often helpful to pass the endoscope through a soft, well-lubricated nasal airway that is spit lengthwise. Once the insertion tube is advanced into the trachea, the airway is removed and the ETT threaded over the insertion tube. Deviation of the nasal septum, which causes lateral displacement of the ETT, is overcome by slight internal rotation of the tube. Retraction of the tongue may facilitate visualization of the larynx by lifting the epiglottis away from the pharynx. Despite the potential for producing bleeding, nasotracheal intubation is often easier than orotracheal intubation because the natural curve of the nasopharynx guides the tube into the larynx.

POSITIONING THE PATIENT

Laryngoscopy is usually performed with the patient in the supine position. When general anesthesia is administered, the endoscopist stands to the left of the assistant, allowing the latter access to the anesthesia machine. Alternatively, the endoscopist may face the patient. Patients who cannot lie flat because of cardiac or pulmonary disease may be intubated in the semi-Fowler's position. Local anesthesia is safest for such patients, and the anesthesiologist faces the patient rather than standing at the head of the table.

ANTICIPATING DIFFICULTY WITH INTUBATION

When difficulty with endotracheal intubation is anticipated on the basis of the patient's anesthetic history or physical examination, it is better to attempt fiberoptic laryngoscopy initially rather than after conventional methods have failed. The patient, surgeon, and operating room personnel must be informed of the potential problems and proposed solutions. Alternatives, including the possibility of tracheostomy, must be discussed prior to the patient's arrival in the operating room. In addition to being available in case a tracheostomy is necessary, the otorhinolaryngologist should be prepared to perform bronchoscopy. He may be able to pass a rigid bronchoscope when fiberoptic endoscopy is impossible. Under these circumstances, the most skilled endoscopist must be present, the surgeon scrubbed, the tracheostomy set open, and the bronchoscope attached to a functional light source. It is essential that the endoscopes and light sources be checked before anesthesia is induced.

Prominent "buck" teeth, a receding mandible and short, thick neck make intubation difficult and are most obvious when the patient is viewed in profile. During the preoperative visit, the patient should be asked to open his mouth and extend his neck so that the physician can detect limited motion of the temporomandibular joints or cervical spine.

If after initial evaluation there is any question regarding the possibility of difficult intubation, the distance between the lower border of the mandible and the thyroid notch should be measured in the midline with the patient's neck fully extended. The normal measurement is 6.5 cm or greater. If the distance is 6.0–6.5 cm, the patient does not have prominent teeth or a small mandible, and the temporomandibular and cervical spine functions are normal, laryngoscopy and intubation are usually possible, but difficult. When the distance is 6.5 cm and one or more of the foregoing abnormalities is present, or the distance is less than 6.0 cm in any patient, it must be presumed that direct laryngoscopy will be impossible and fiberoptic laryngoscopy is indicated.

UNPREDICTED DIFFICULTY WITH ENDOTRACHEAL INTUBATION

It is not always possible to predict that endotracheal intubation will be difficult. Managing such patients is a humbling and challenging experience for the anesthesiologist. Often there are better solutions than fiberoptic endoscopy. The alternatives must be discussed with the surgeon and agreement reached. If the procedure is elective, multiple intubation attempts have resulted in trauma, and there is no skilled fiberoptic endoscopist available, the solution is simple: terminate the procedure.

If the difficulty is recognized before trauma is produced, the patient is in stable condition, and an experienced fiberoptic endoscopist and appropriate equipment are available, it is reasonable to proceed. General anesthesia is continued. If a depolarizing muscle relaxant was administered, it is allowed to wear off. A nondepolarizing relaxant is reversed. Atropine should be administered for its drying effect as soon as the decision is made to proceed. If the esophagus has been intubated or positive-pressure ventilation has resulted in distention of the stomach, a nasogastric tube is inserted and the stomach decompressed. The spontaneously breathing patient is then intubated with the help of an endoscopic mask and airway.

When the procedure is emergent and the patient's condition is unstable, general anesthesia is abandoned and the patient allowed to awaken. If fiberoptic endoscopy is attempted and the patient has a full stomach, topical anesthesia and sedatives should be used with caution, if at all. In these circumstances a transtracheal block should never be performed. The most conservative and safest approach is to avoid all local anesthetics because it is impossible to insure that topical anesthesia will be confined to the area above the vocal cords, and aspiration is a very real danger.

The patient whose condition is deteriorating as a result of cardiovascular instability or respiratory obstruction is almost never a candidate for fiberoptic endoscopy. Only if the equipment is immediately available and a skilled endoscopist is in attendance should it be considered. Cricothyrotomy, rigid bronchoscopy, or tracheostomy is preferable.

COMPLICATIONS AND PRECAUTIONS

The complications are the same as with conventional laryngoscopy and include tissue trauma, bleeding, and laryngospasm. In the awake patient, gagging can be reduced with adequate topical anesthesia, and coughing is minimized by a transtracheal block. However, these techniques should not be used in the patient with a full stomach because of the danger of aspiration.

If the principles listed in Tables 5–1 and 5–2 are followed, fiberoptic laryngoscopy is more likely to be successful and accomplished with minimal trauma.

TABLE 5–1.—FIBEROPTIC LARYNGOSCOPY FOR ENDOTRACHEAL INTUBATION

Check endoscope and light source
Apply antifog agent to lens
Focus lens prior to use
Lubricate insertion tube (avoid lens)
Remove connector of ETT and cut tube to correct length
Insert endoscope into ETT
Introduce endoscope into pharynx, maintain in midline, and advance 8–10 cm
Look into endoscope and identify structures
Flex tip of endoscope upward to visualize larynx
Rotate distal end of insertion tube toward midline if necessary
Enter vocal cords, return tip of endoscope to neutral position, and advance
Position endoscope just above carina and thread ETT

TABLE 5–2.—GUIDELINES FOR FIBEROPTIC LARYNGOSCOPY IN THE PATIENT WITH A DIFFICULT AIRWAY

Discuss the problems and formulate a plan with the surgeon
Administer an antisialagogue preoperatively
Employ fiberoptic endoscopy initially when difficulty is anticipated
Use equipment with which you are most familiar
Have available conventional laryngoscopes with various blades, resuscitation equipment, cricothyrotomy needle, a tracheostomy set, rigid bronchoscopes, and light sources
Ascertain that the endoscope and light sources are functional
Induce anesthesia only after all equipment and personnel are prepared
Allow sufficient time for anesthesia
Arrange for an assistant to monitor patient
Ask for help from another endoscopist when needed

GAINING FACILITY WITH THE INSTRUMENT

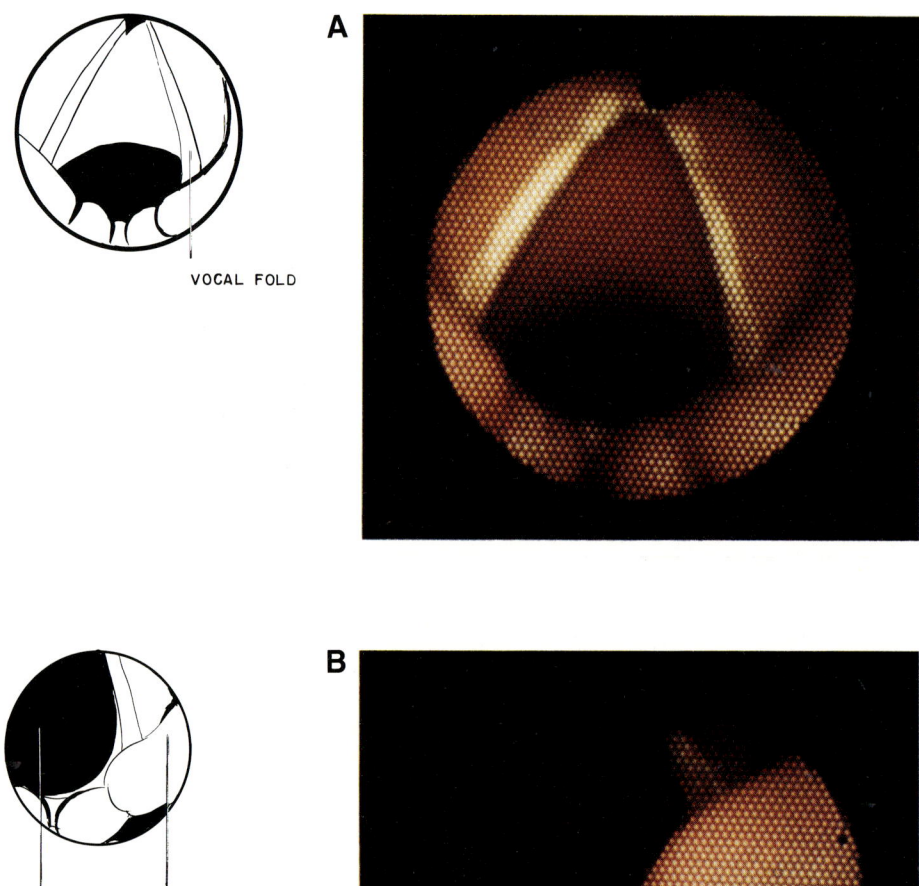

Fig 5–1.—The endoscopic appearance of the larynx **(A)** and the aryepiglottic folds **(B)** in the mannequin. Endoscopic intubation is best learned step-by-step on a mannequin. This allows practice in manipulating and operating the endoscope without concern for patient safety.

PREPARATION OF EQUIPMENT

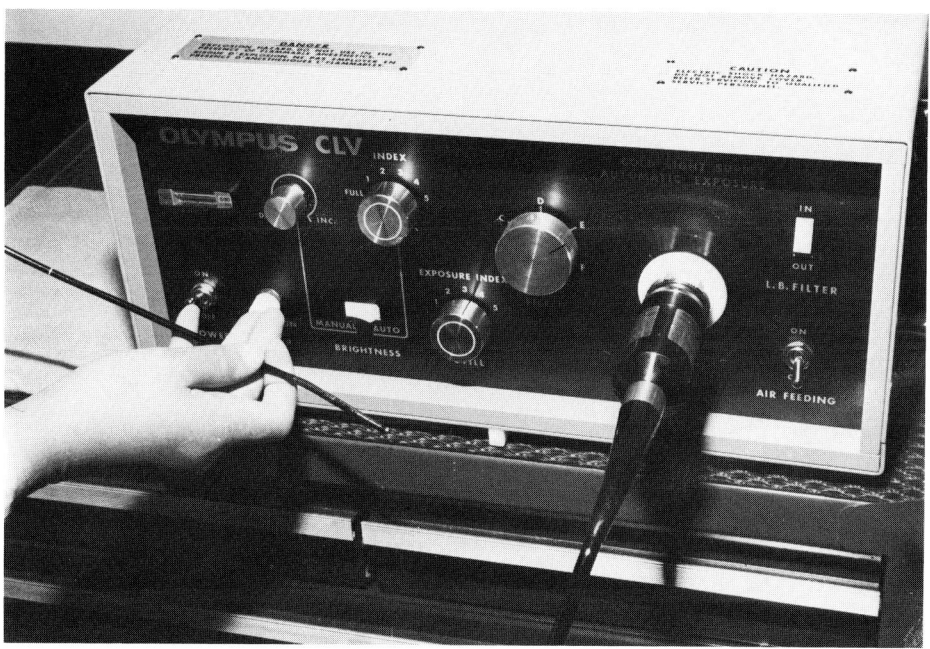

Fig 5–2.—Electrical connections and light intensity must be verified before proceeding.

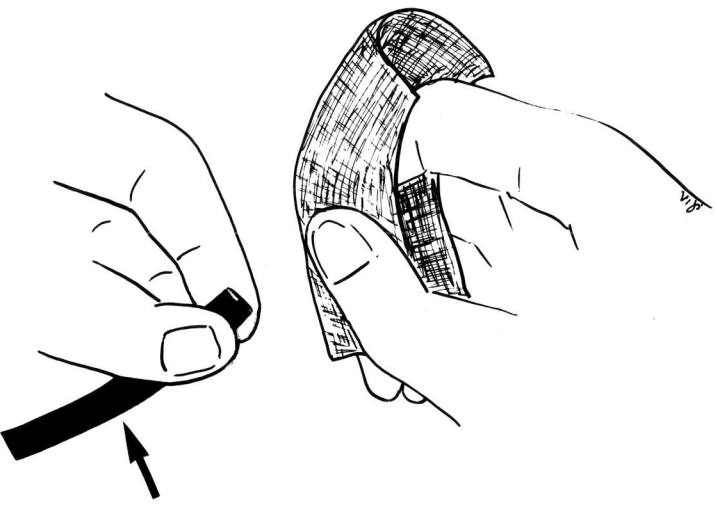

Fig 5–3.—Defogging soap is applied to the lens. The distal tip is held beyond the angle bend joint *(arrow)* to avoid damage to the fibers and to the angle bend mechanism.

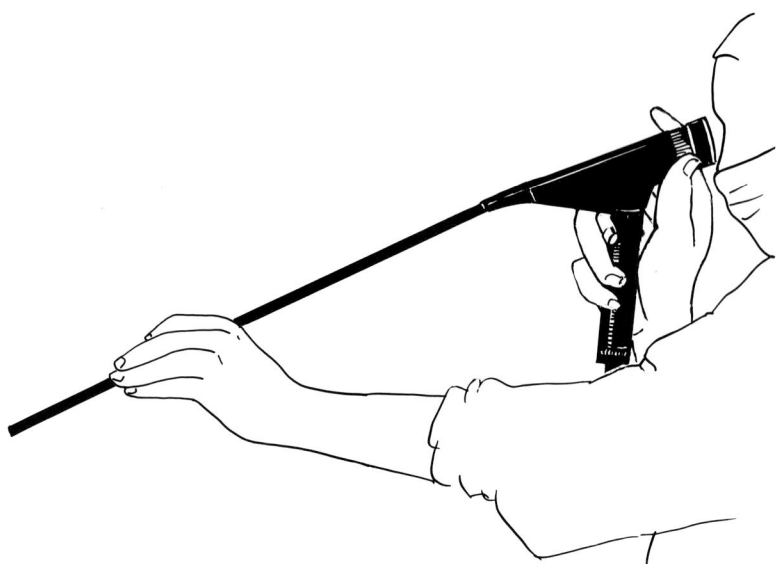

Fig 5–4.—The lens must be focused before insertion. Precise focusing is best achieved by focusing on a lettered object. The focus should not be adjusted after introduction of the insertion tube.

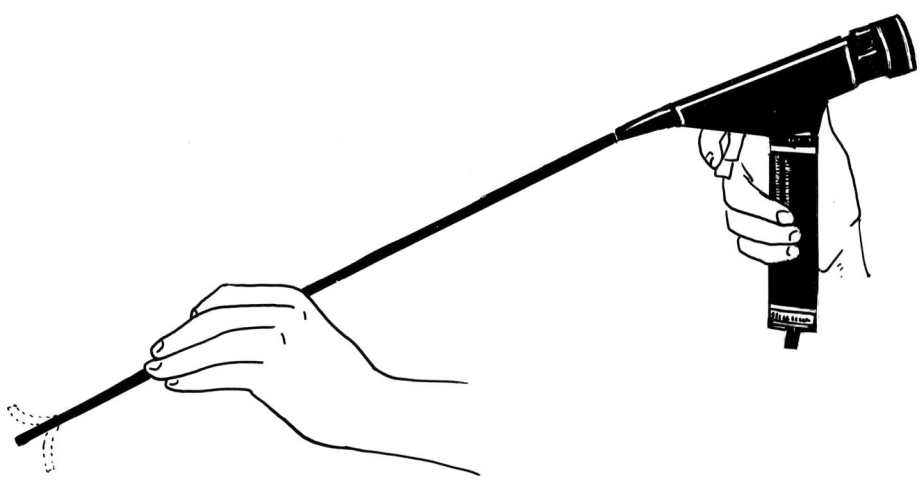

Fig 5–5.—The bending angle is checked before threading the ETT.

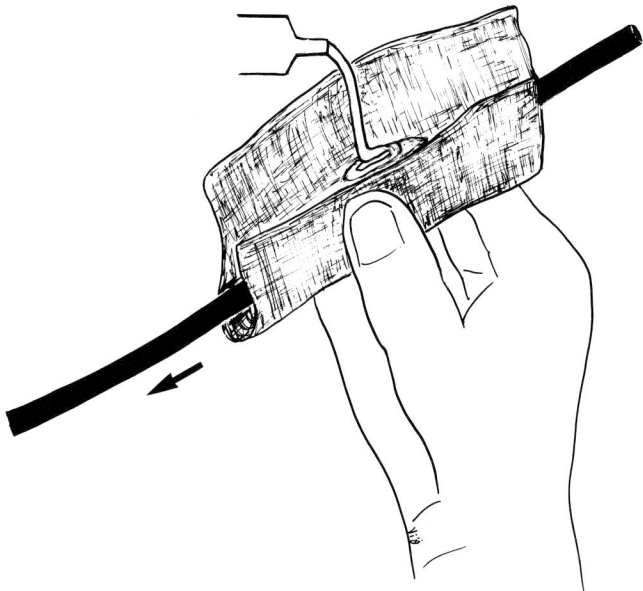

Fig 5–6.—Lubricant is applied only in a distal-to-proximal manner to avoid obscuring the lens.

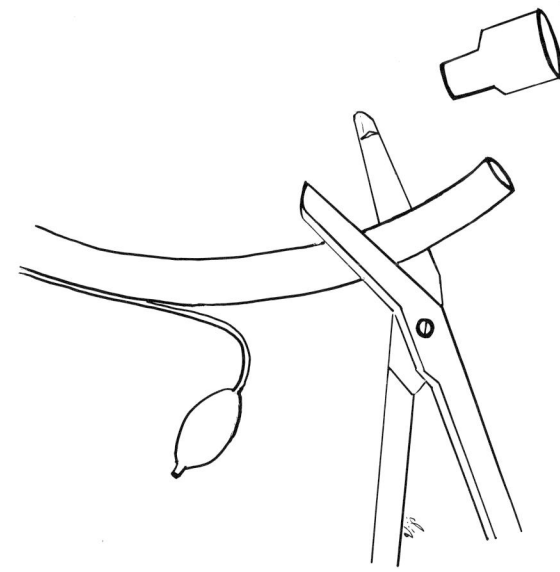

Fig 5–7.—The ETT is cut to the appropriate length.

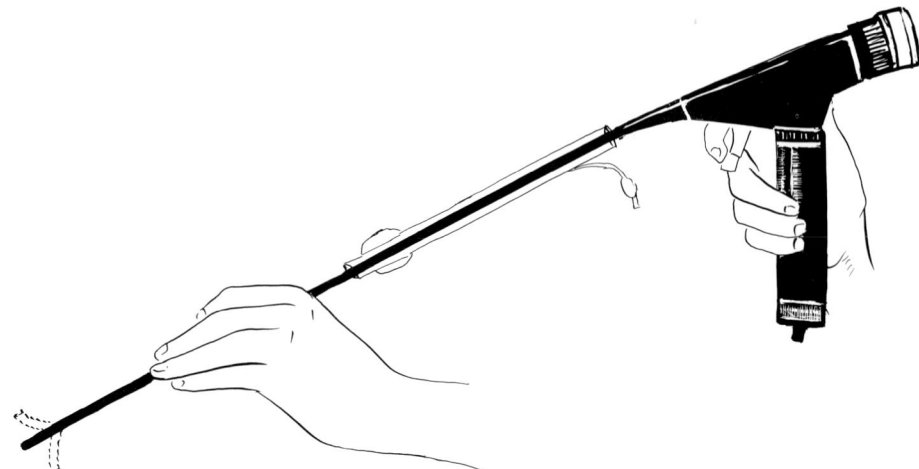

Fig 5–8.—The ETT, without a connector, is threaded over the insertion tube. The direction of the endoscope tip is again verified to be in a vertical plane.

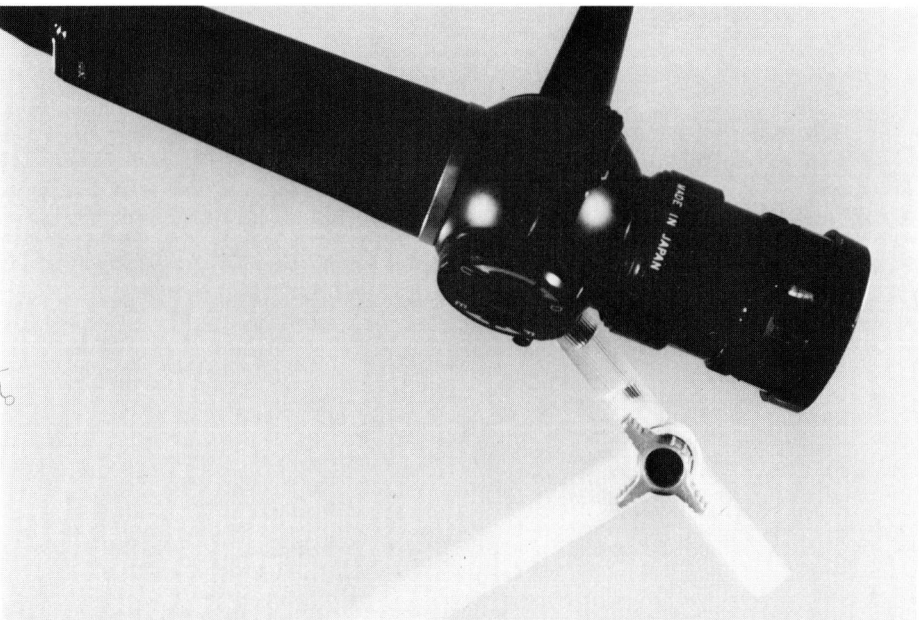

Fig 5–9.—The operating channel is connected to suction. A three-way stopcock is placed to alternate suctioning with oxygen administration.

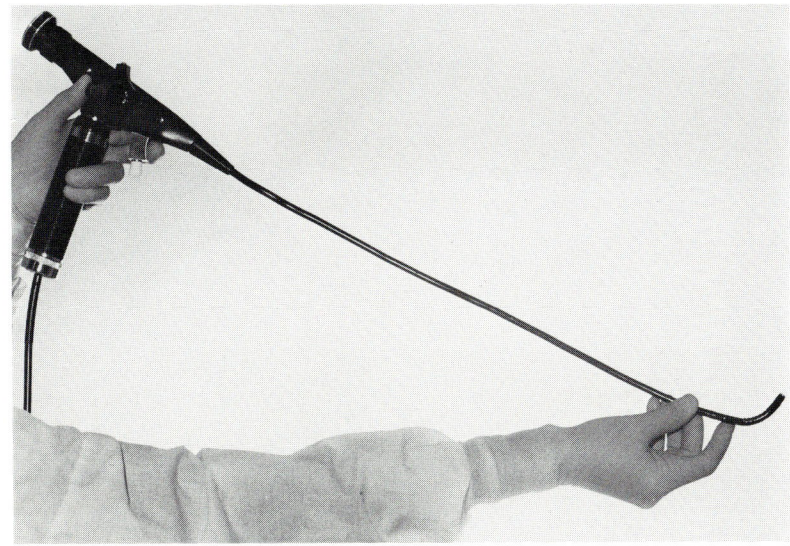

Fig 5–10.—The control section is held with one hand by placing the thumb on the angle bend knob and the index finger on the suction port.

PLACEMENT OF THE INSERTION TUBE

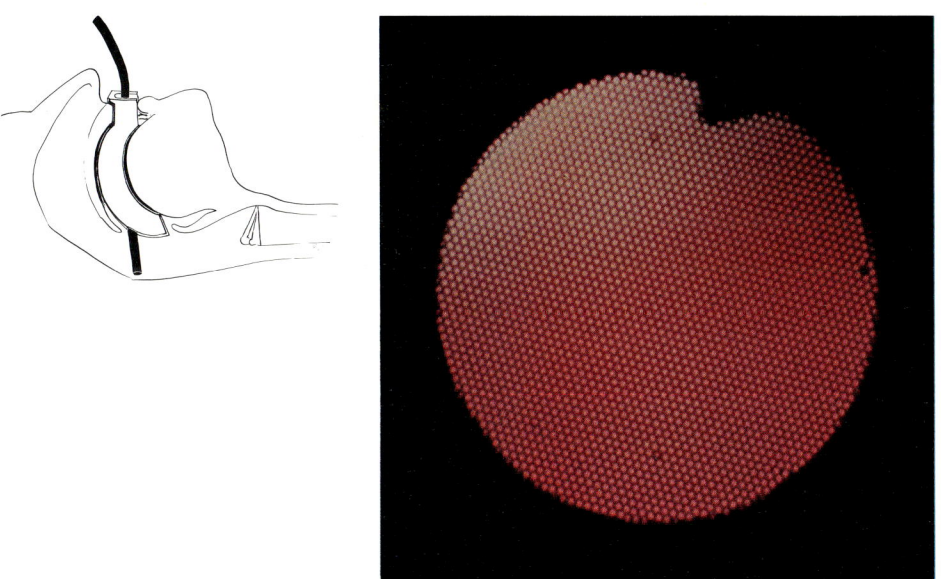

Fig 5–11.—The insertion tube is introduced 8–10 cm in the midline, preferably using an endoscopic airway, and the pharynx is visualized.

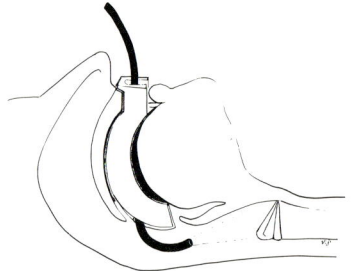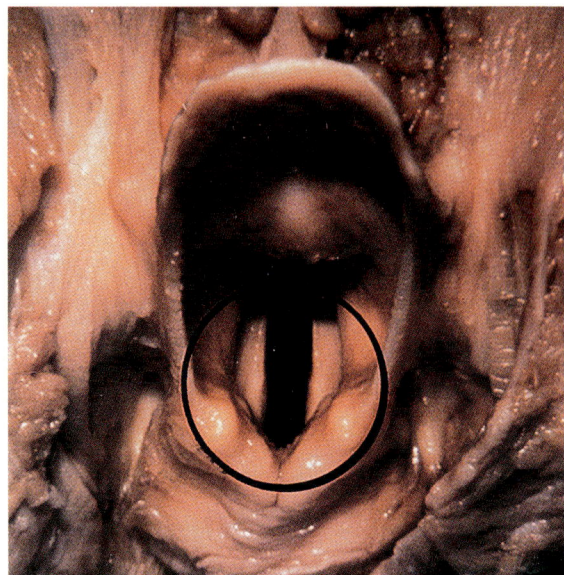

Fig 5–12.

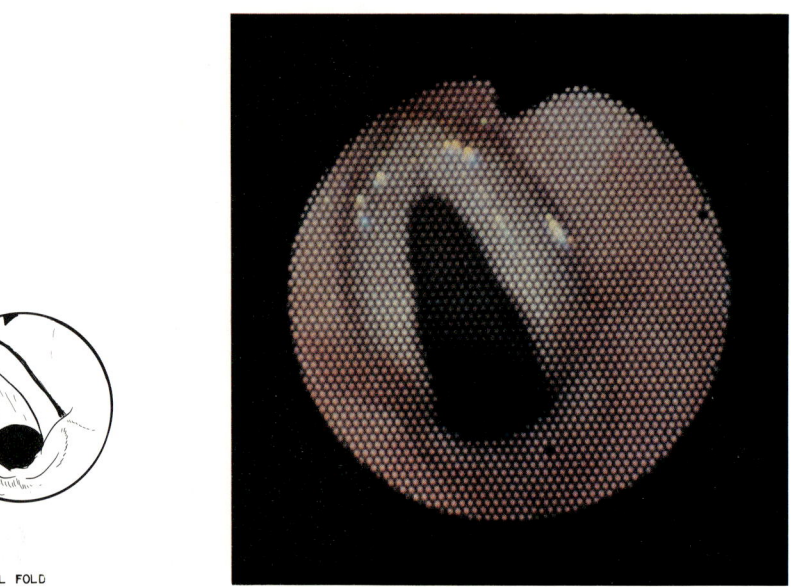

Fig 5–12.—The distal tip is angled anteriorly, using the angle bend knob to visualize the larynx.

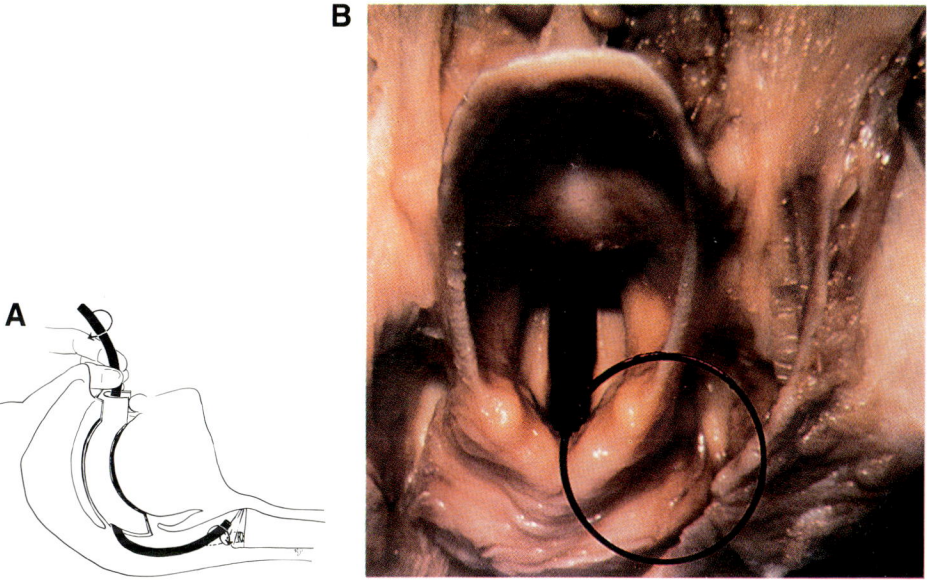

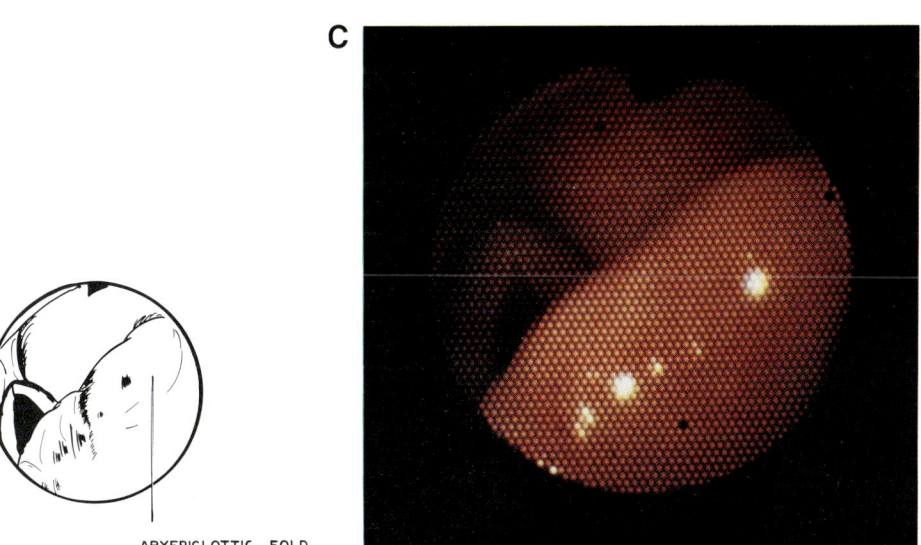

ARYEPIGLOTTIC FOLD

Fig 5–13.—**A,** If the tip of the insertion tube is not in the midline, slight internal rotation of the insertion tube will guide the tip into the midline. **B, C,** structures seen when the insertion tube is not in the midline. **D, E,** view after internal rotation of the insertion tube.

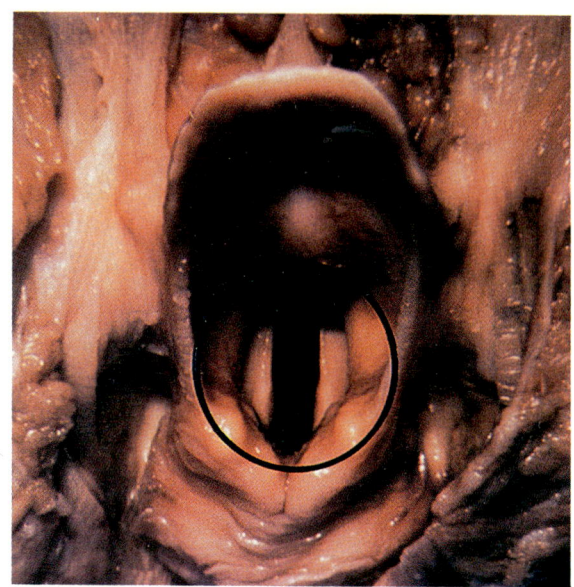

Fig 5–13 D.

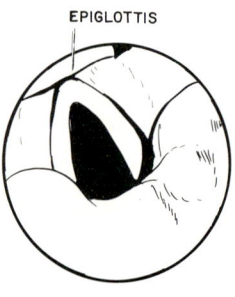

Fig 5–13 E.

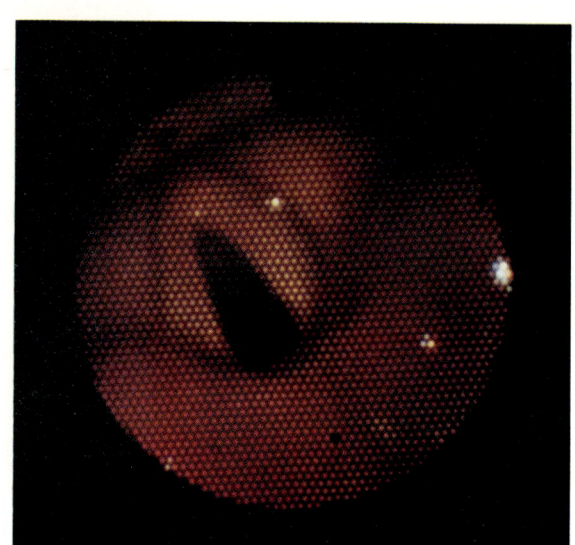

Fig 5–14 A.

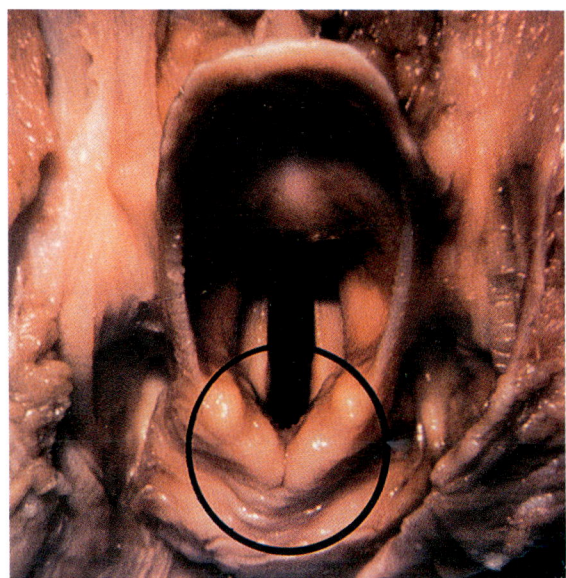

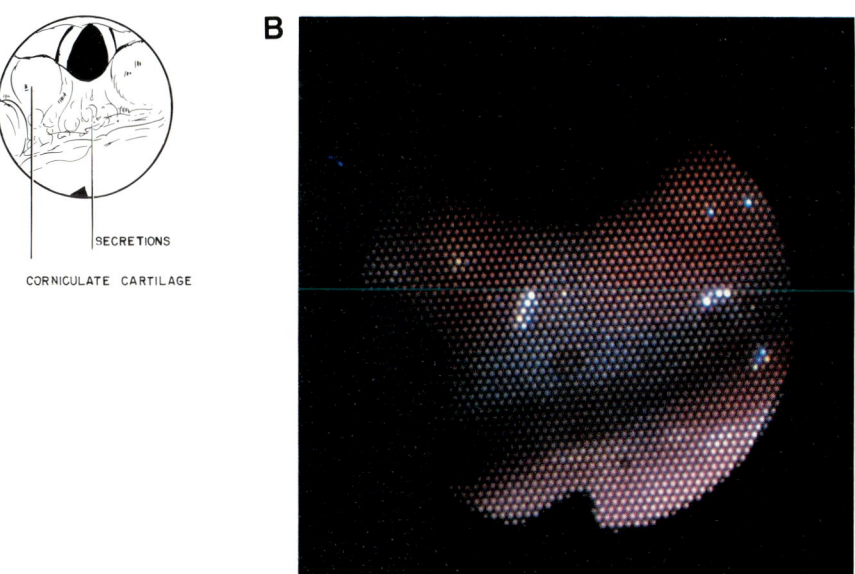

Fig 5–14.—**A, B,** structures seen when the insertion tube is angled too far posteriorly. **C, D,** view after the insertion tube is angled anteriorly.

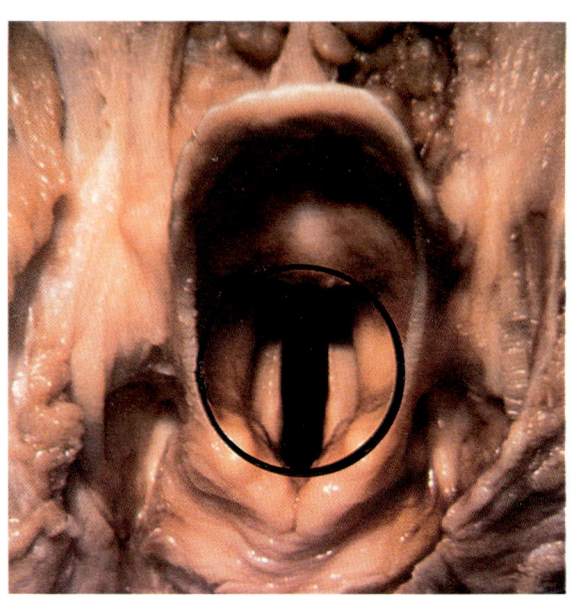

Fig 5–14 C.

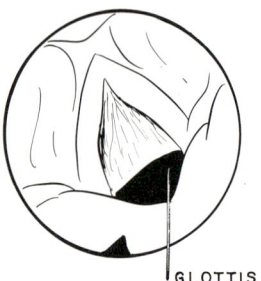

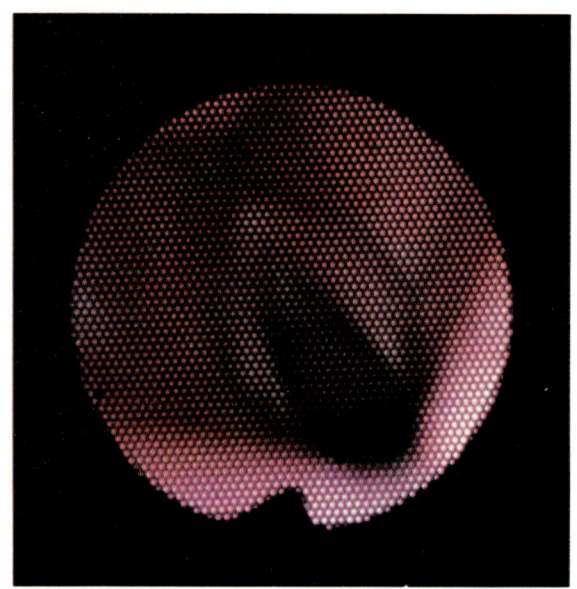

Fig 5–14 D.

Fig 5–15 A.

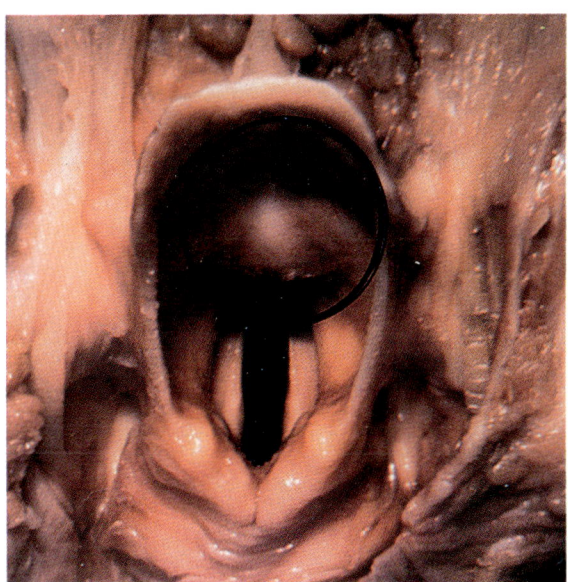

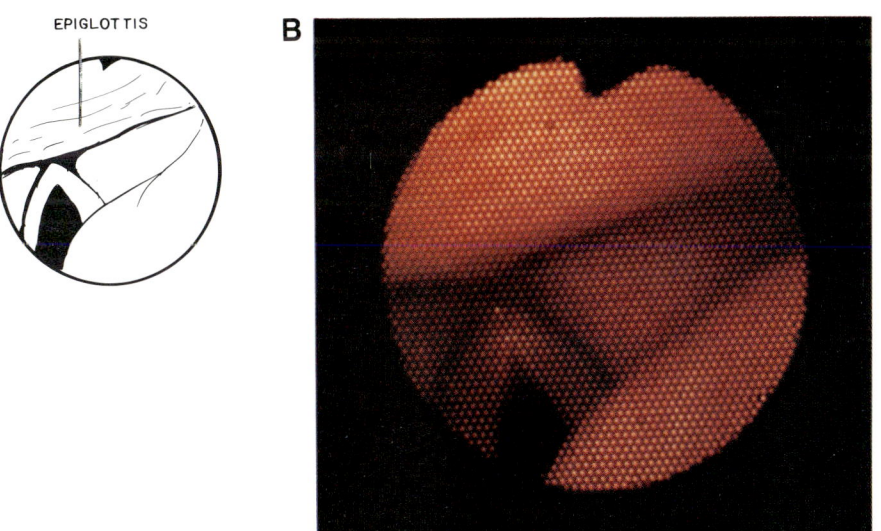

Fig 5–15.—**A, B,** structures seen when the insertion tube is angled too far anteriorly. **C, D,** view after the tube is angled posteriorly.

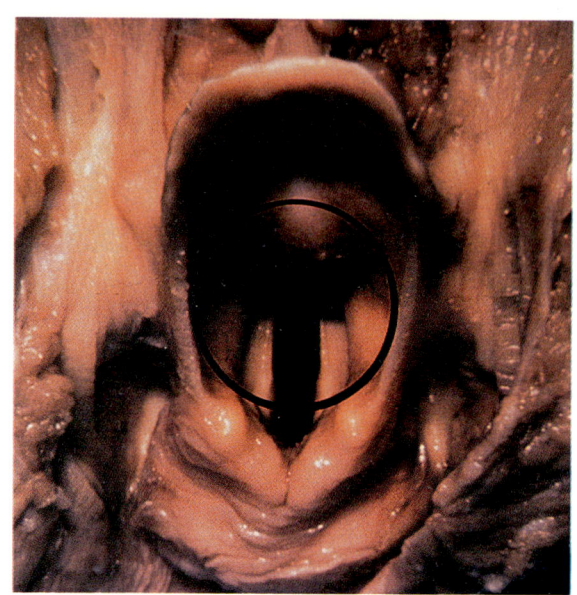

Fig 5–15 C.

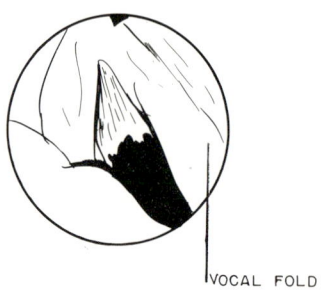

VOCAL FOLD

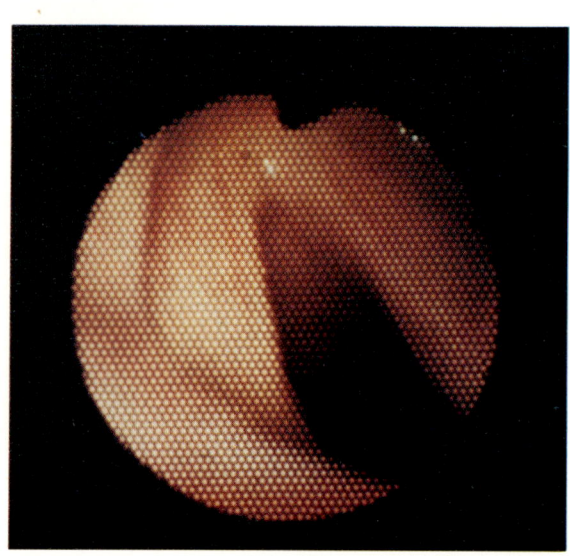

Fig 5–15 D.

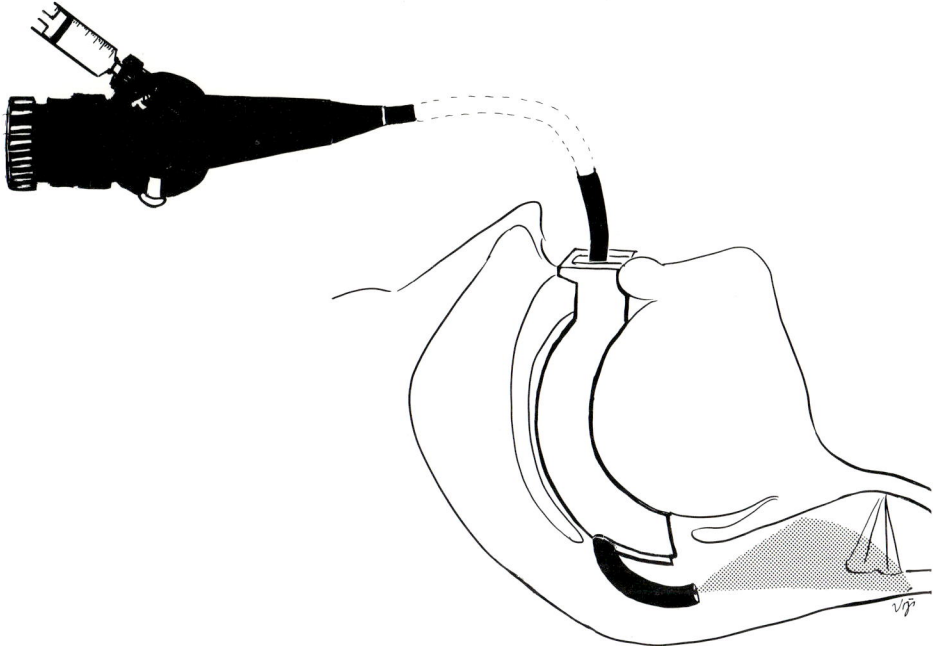

Fig 5–16.—A local anesthetic agent can be instilled through the operating channel if the vocal cords are moving and topical anesthesia is inadequate.

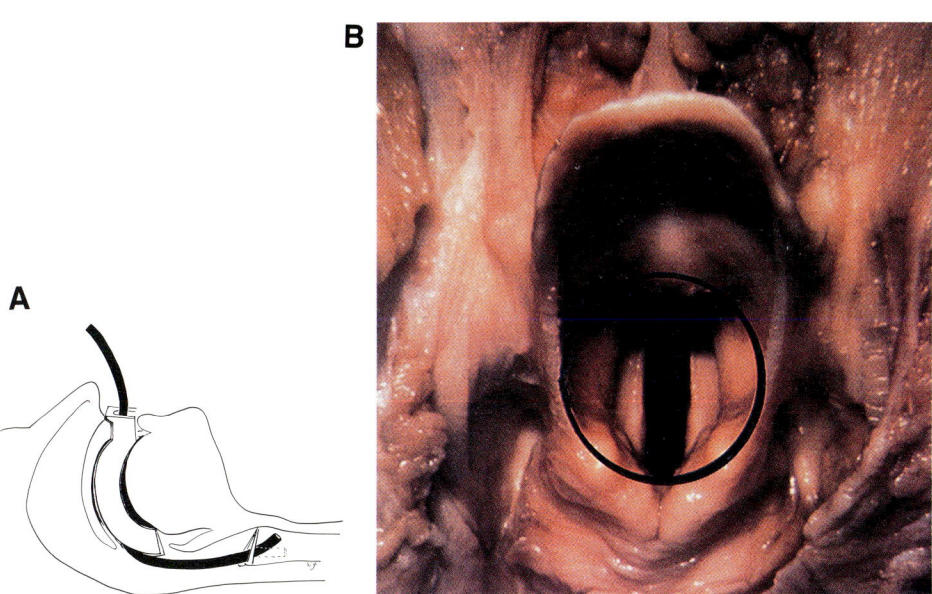

Fig 5–17.—**A, B, C,** the glottis is entered with the tip of the insertion tube angled slightly upward, bringing the thyroid and cricoid cartilages into view. If the larynx is very anterior, it is necessary to reduce the angle of the tip of the insertion tube prior to entering the larynx.

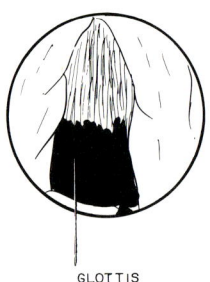
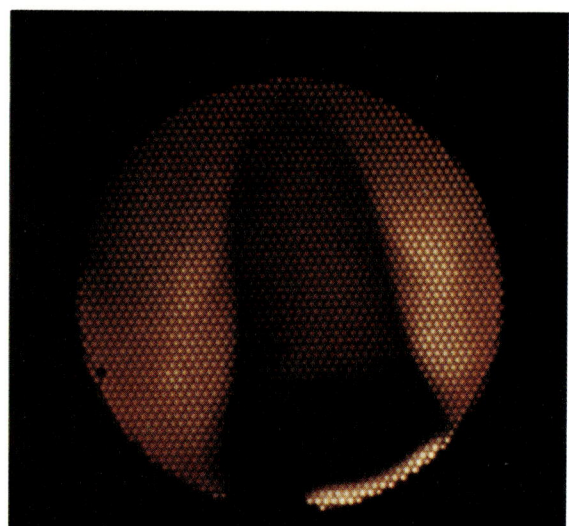

Fig 5–17 C.

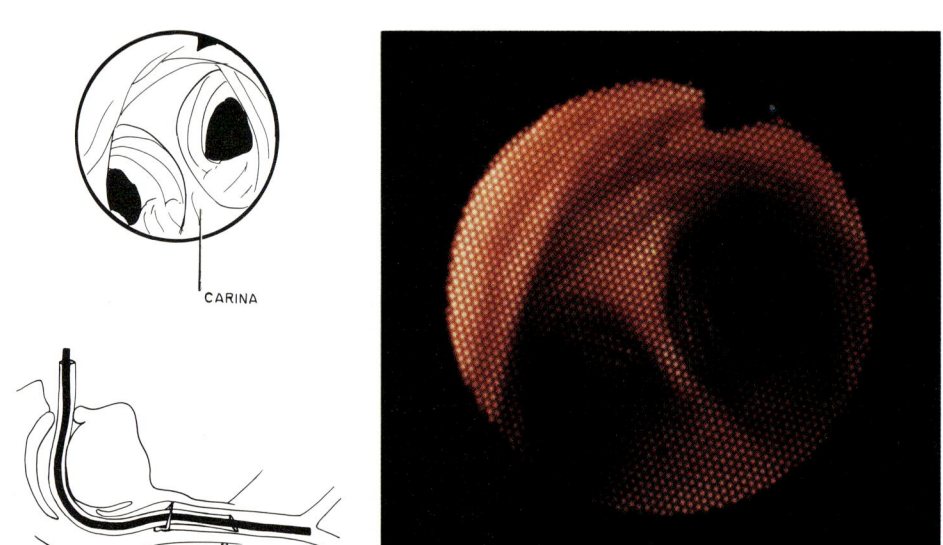

Fig 5–18.—The tip of the insertion tube is straightened as it is advanced, bringing the tracheal cartilages into view. The insertion tube is advanced until the tip lies just above the carina. The ETT is threaded over the insertion tube, and the endoscope is removed.

REASONS FOR FAILURE

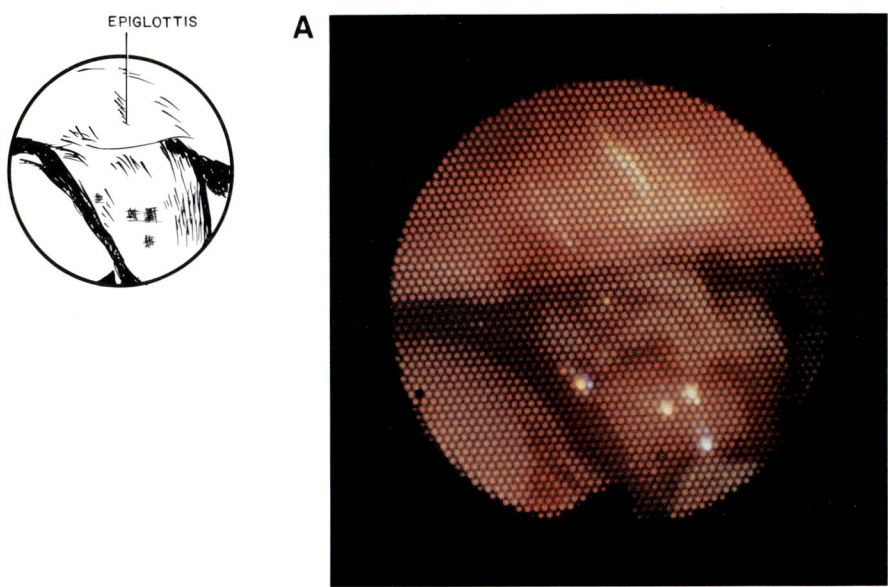

Fig 5–19.—Bleeding resulting from previous attempts at intubation **(A–C)**. Secretions **(D)**. Lens not focused **(E)**. Lens not defogged **(F)**. Insufficient light **(G)**. Broken fibers **(H)**.

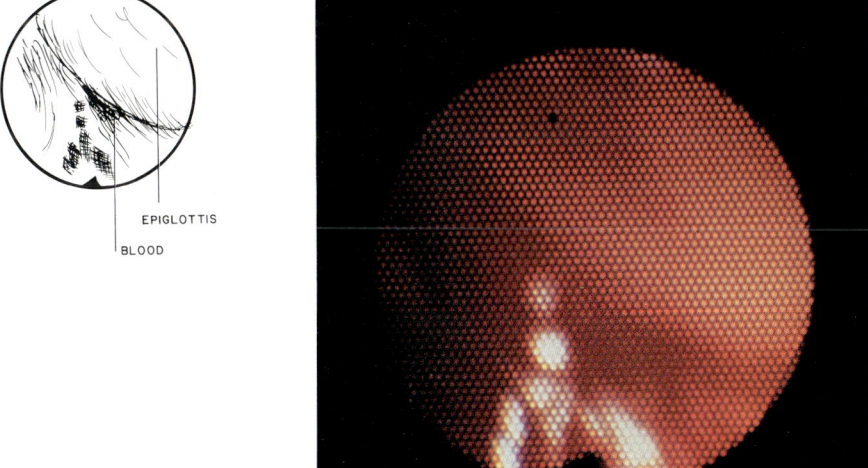

Fig 5–19 B.

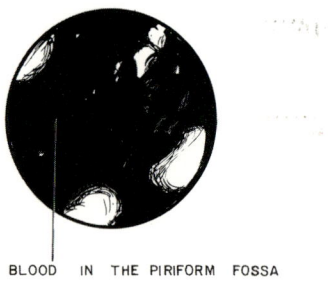
BLOOD IN THE PIRIFORM FOSSA

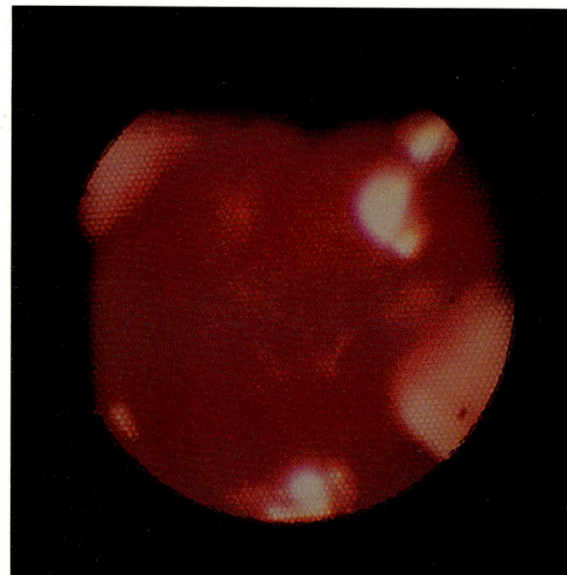

Fig 5–19 C.

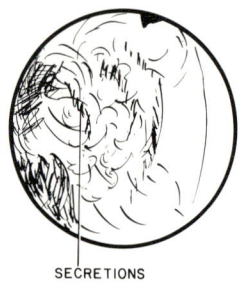
SECRETIONS

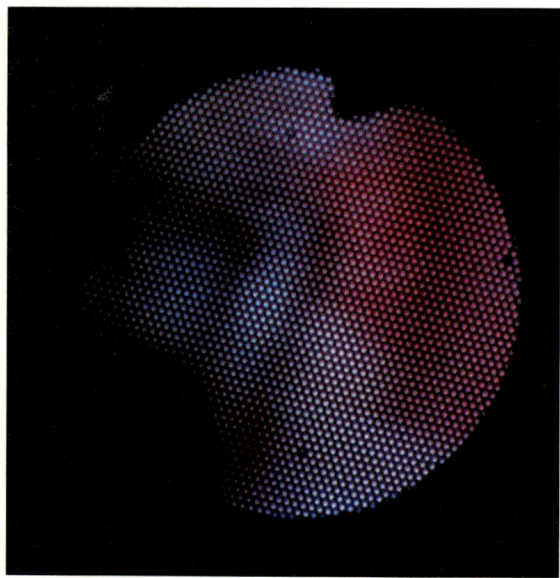

Fig 5–19 D.

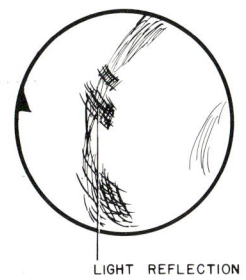
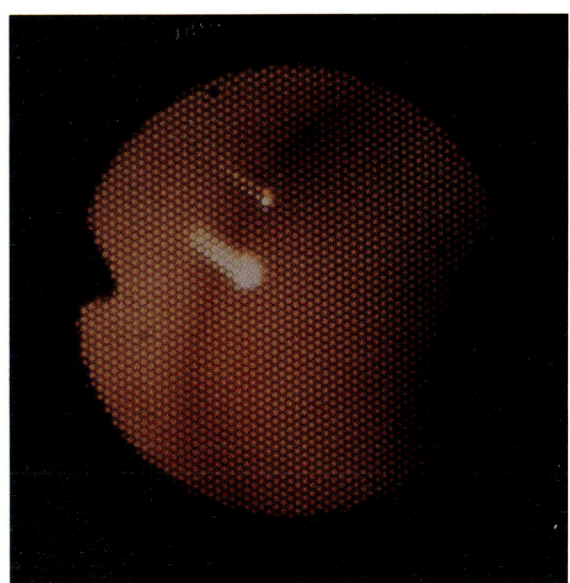

Fig 5–19 E.

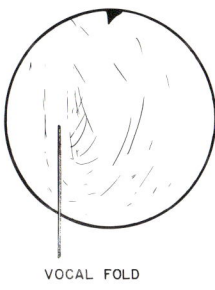
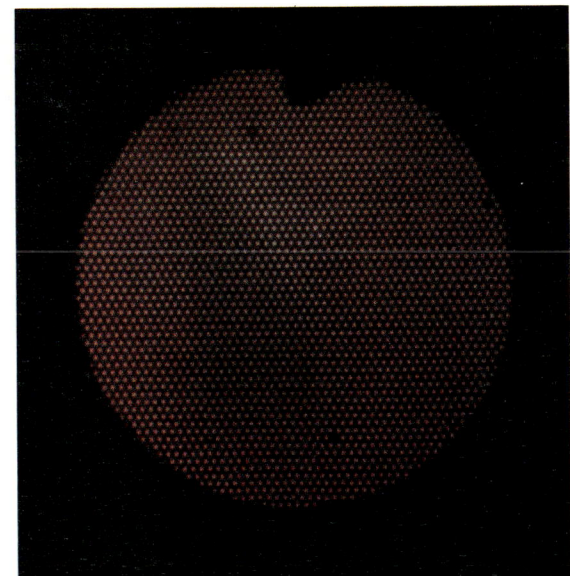

Fig 5–19 F.

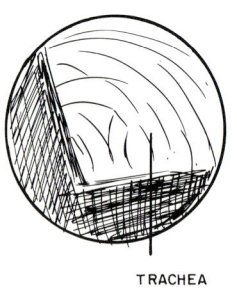
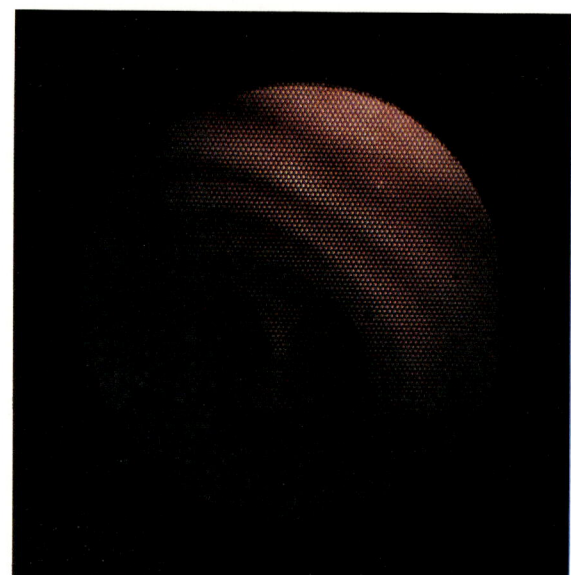

Fig 5–19 G.

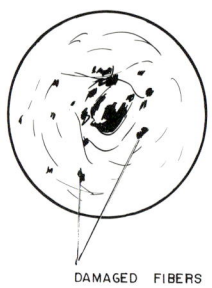
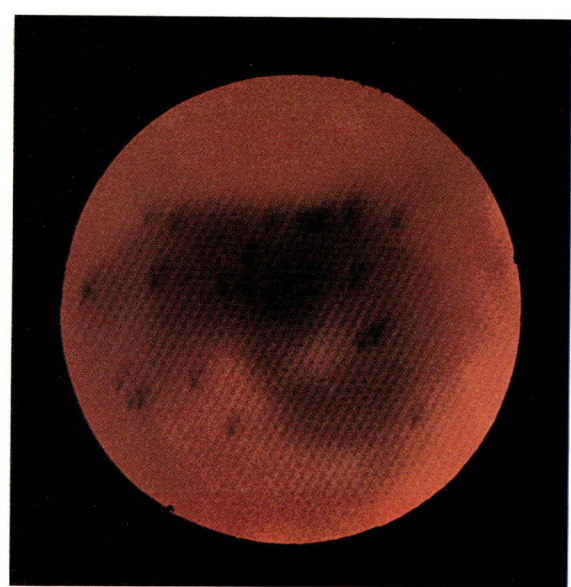

Fig 5–19 H.

NERVE BLOCK TECHNIQUES

Internal Laryngeal Nerve Block

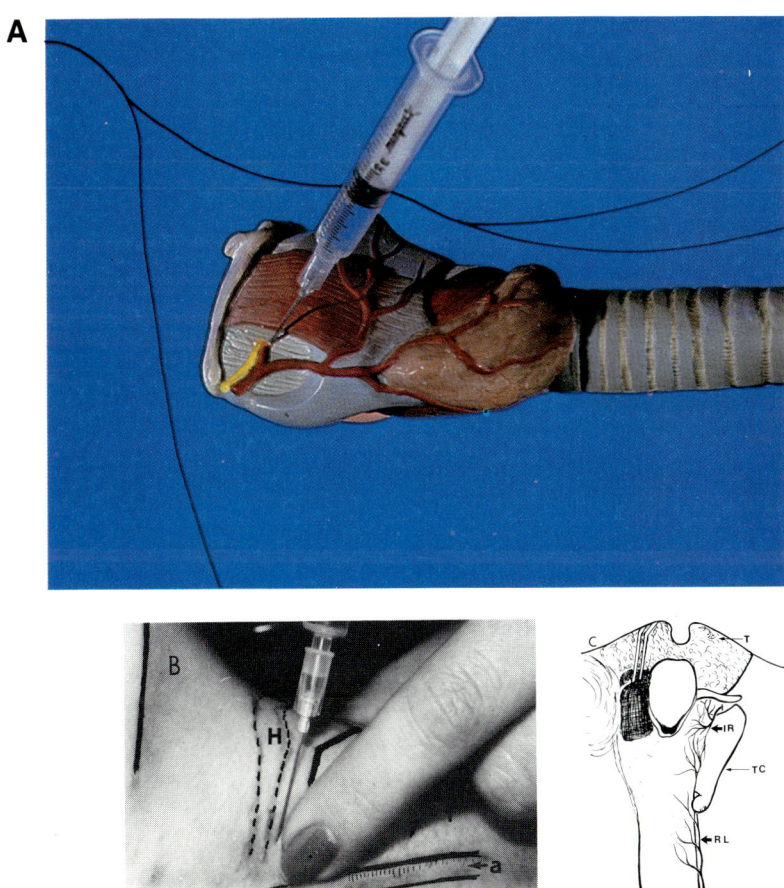

Fig 5–20.—The internal laryngeal nerve, a branch of the superior laryngeal nerve, pierces the thyrohyoid membrane just inferior to the greater cornu of the hyoid bone **(A)**. Applying pressure to the opposite greater cornu displaces the laryngeal structures to the side to be blocked and facilitates identification of anatomical landmarks. After cleansing the skin with alcohol, 3 ml of 2% lidocaine is injected at the level of the thyrohyoid membrane, using a 25-gauge needle directed cephalad and medially **(B)**. If air is aspirated, indicating that the pharynx has been entered, the needle is withdrawn slightly prior to injection of the anesthetic. Bilateral nerve blocks will produce anesthesia over the inferior aspect of the epiglottis and the laryngeal outlet above the vocal folds. The nerve can also be blocked by placing a sponge saturated with local anesthetic in the piriform fossa **(C)**. The sponge should remain in contact with the tissue for 3–5 minutes. T = posterior surface of the tongue; IR = internal laryngeal nerve; TC = thyroid cartilage; and RL = recurrent laryngeal nerve.

Transtracheal Block

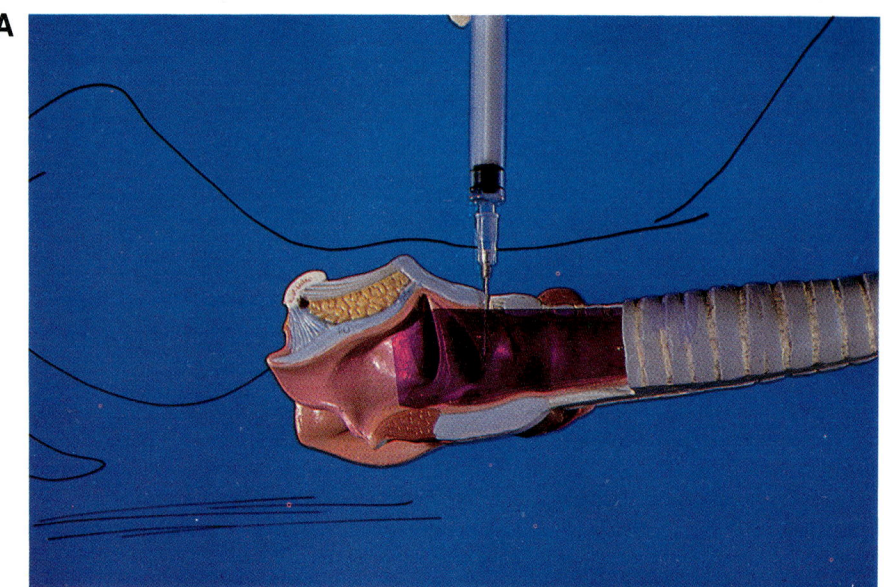

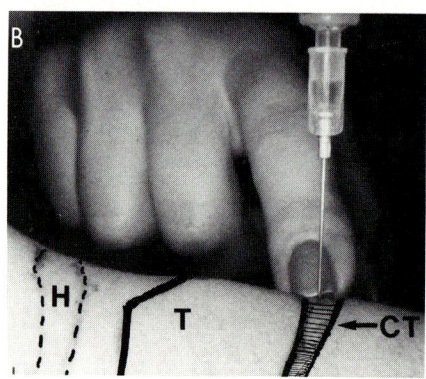

Fig 5–21.—Anesthesia below the vocal folds *(shaded area,* **A***)* is achieved by transtracheal instillation of local anesthetics. With the patient's neck in full extension **(B)**, the cricothyroid membrane (CT) is palpated in the midline as a slight depression between the lower border of the thyroid cartilage (T) and the cricoid cartilage. The area is cleansed with alcohol and a 22-gauge needle introduced perpendicular to the skin. After air is aspirated from the trachea, 3–5 ml of 2% lidocaine is injected. The needle is removed immediately because the patient will cough vigorously. Pressure is applied over the injected area to prevent hematoma formation.

ENDOSCOPIC INTUBATION UNDER GENERAL ANESTHESIA

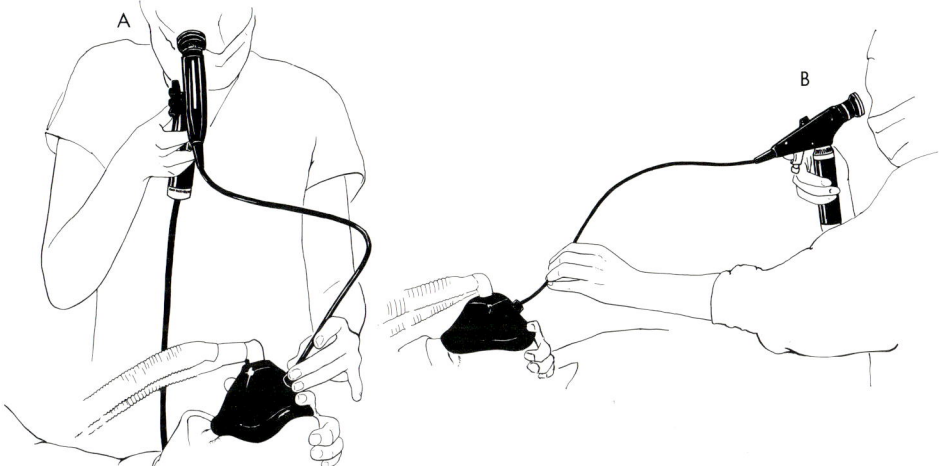

Fig 5–22.—The presence of an assistant is essential when performing endoscopic intubation with general anesthesia. **A,** the endoscopist usually stands at the head of the patient and to the left of the assistant to allow the latter access to the anesthesia machine and monitoring equipment. **B,** alternatively, the endoscopist may stand facing the patient.

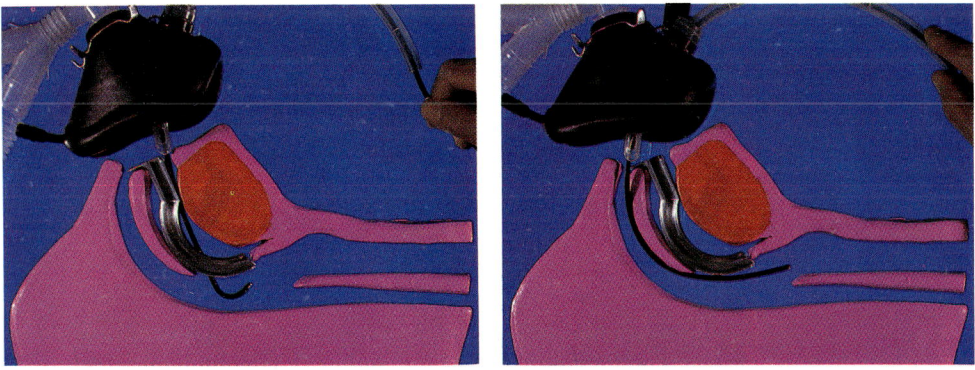

Fig 5–23.—Fiberoptic endoscopy in the anesthetized patient is facilitated by the Patil-Syracuse mask and airway. *Left,* orotracheal intubation; *right,* nasotracheal intubation.

Orotracheal Intubation

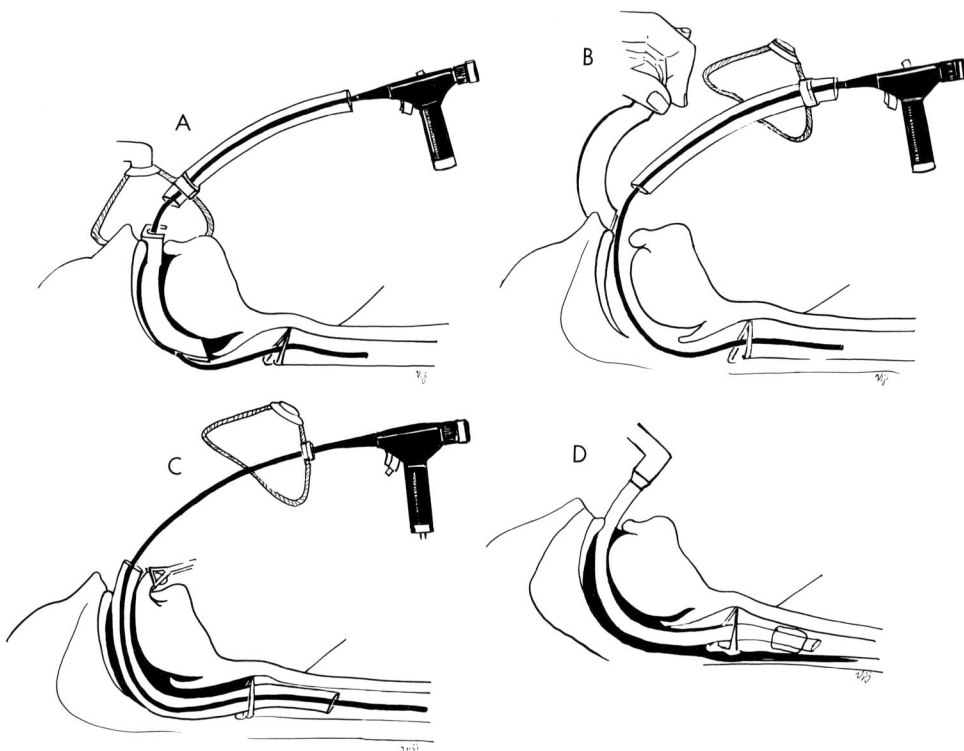

Fig 5-24.—The insertion tube and the ETT are introduced through the port of the endoscopic mask and the insertion tube is advanced to a level just above the carina **(A).** The ETT is advanced through the mask as the latter and the endoscopic airway are removed **(B).** The ETT is advanced through the vocal cords. If difficulty is encountered, it may be necessary to pull the tongue forward with a tongue holder. The ETT is held in place while the endoscope and mask are removed **(C)** and the ETT connector is inserted for attachment to the anesthetic circuit **(D).**

Nasotracheal Intubation

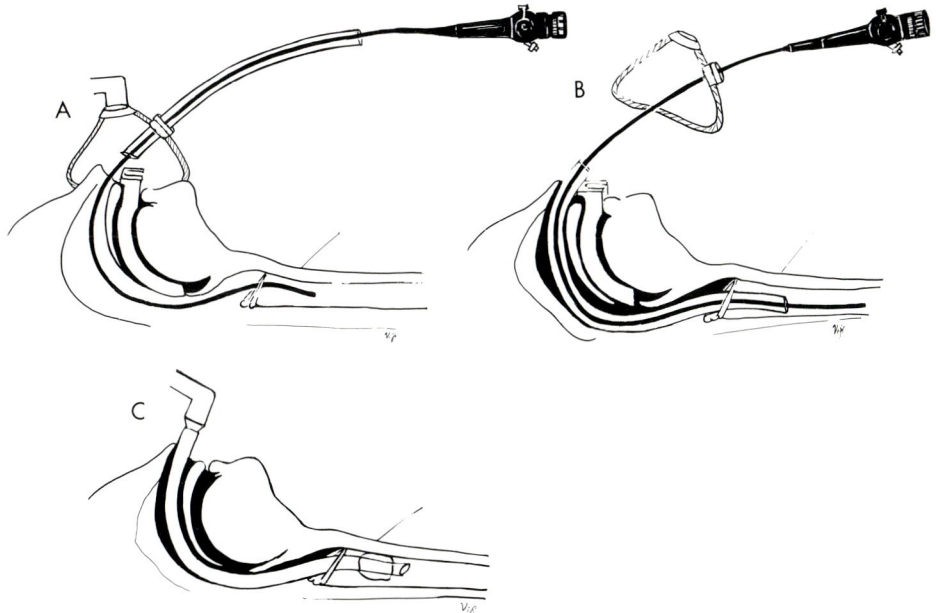

Fig 5–25.—With the endoscopic airway placed to retract the tongue, the insertion tube and ETT are inserted through the port of the endoscopic mask. The insertion tube is advanced through the nose and positioned just above the carina **(A)**. The ETT is drawn through the mask, advanced over the insertion tube and positioned in the trachea **(B)**. The mask and endoscope are removed, and the ETT is connected to the anesthetic circuit **(C)**.

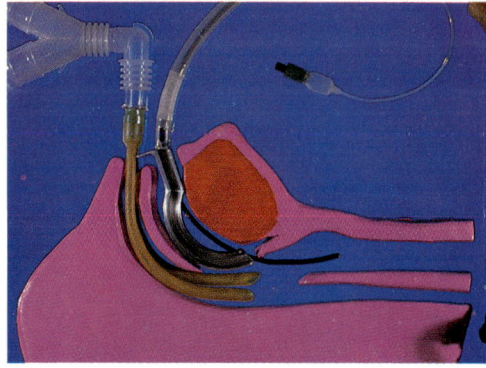

Fig 5–26.—When a binasal airway is used, an endoscopic airway should also be placed for retraction of the tongue and maintenance of the midline position of the insertion tube during orotracheal intubation. The endoscopic airway must be removed prior to advancement of the ETT if the ETT diameter is larger than the central groove of the airway.

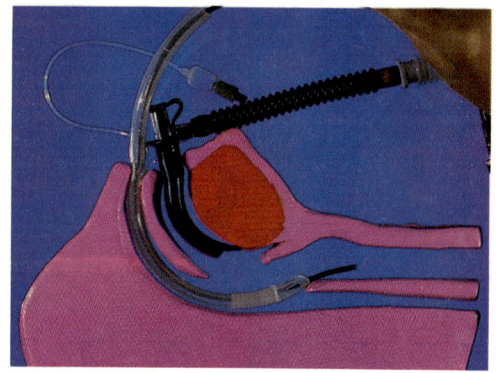

Fig 5–27.—Nasotracheal intubation can be performed utilizing an oral airway with a right-angle connector. Suctioning can be performed through the suction port without interrupting endoscopy.

ENDOSCOPIC INTUBATION WITH LOCAL ANESTHESIA

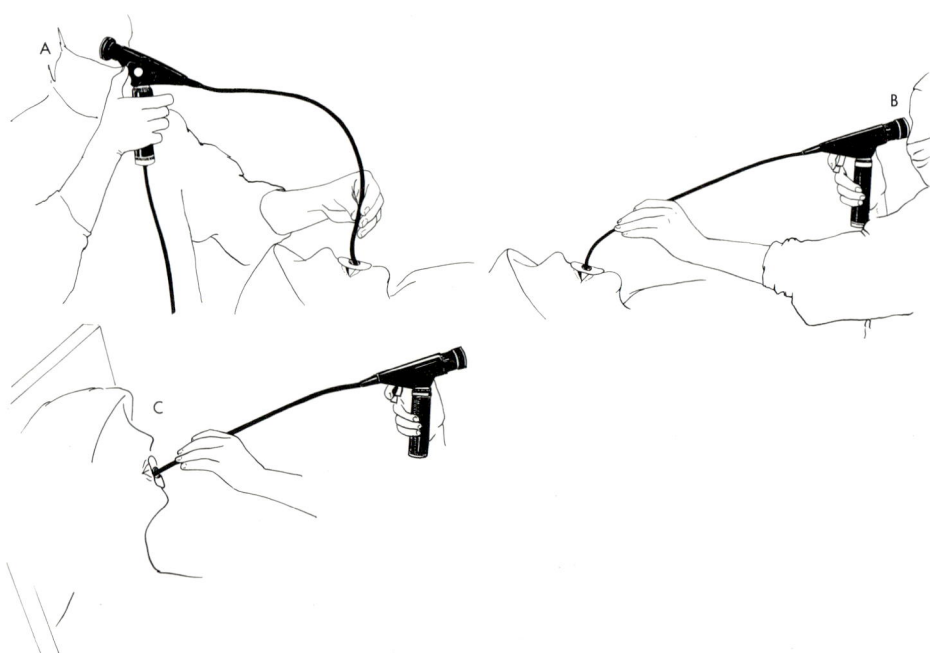

Fig 5–28.—The endoscopist stands at the head of the patient **(A)** or facing the patient **(B)**, according to his preference. When the patient is unable to lie flat, endoscopy can be performed with local anesthesia with the patient in the sitting position **(C)**.

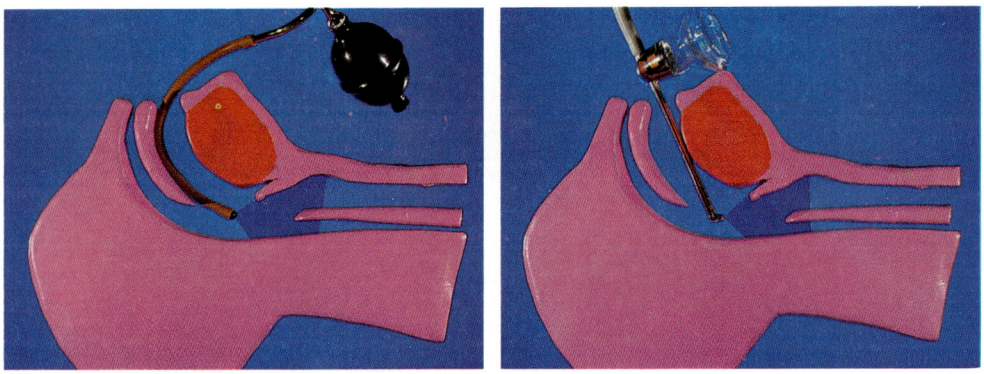

Fig 5–29.—The hypopharynx, oropharynx, and subglottic areas can be anesthetized by applying a local anesthetic agent with an atomizer.

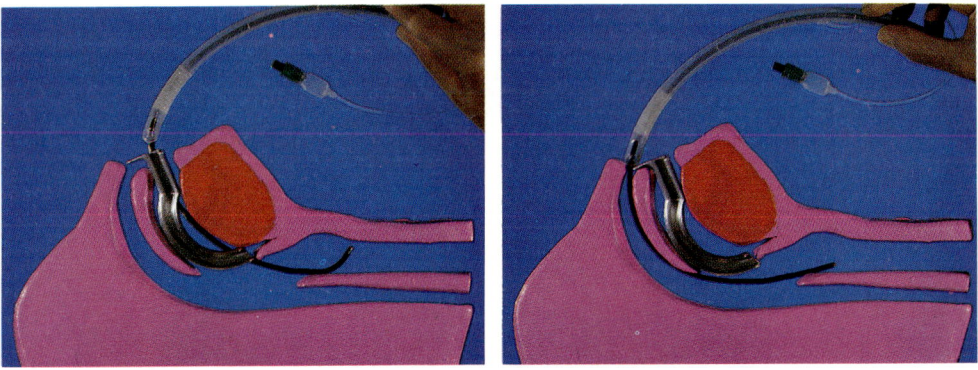

Fig 5–30.—The endoscopic airway is useful during orotracheal intubation with local anesthesia to guide the insertion tube in the midline and to prevent the patient from biting the insertion tube *(left)*. The airway is used to retract the tongue from the pharynx during endoscopic nasotracheal intubation with local anesthesia *(right)*.

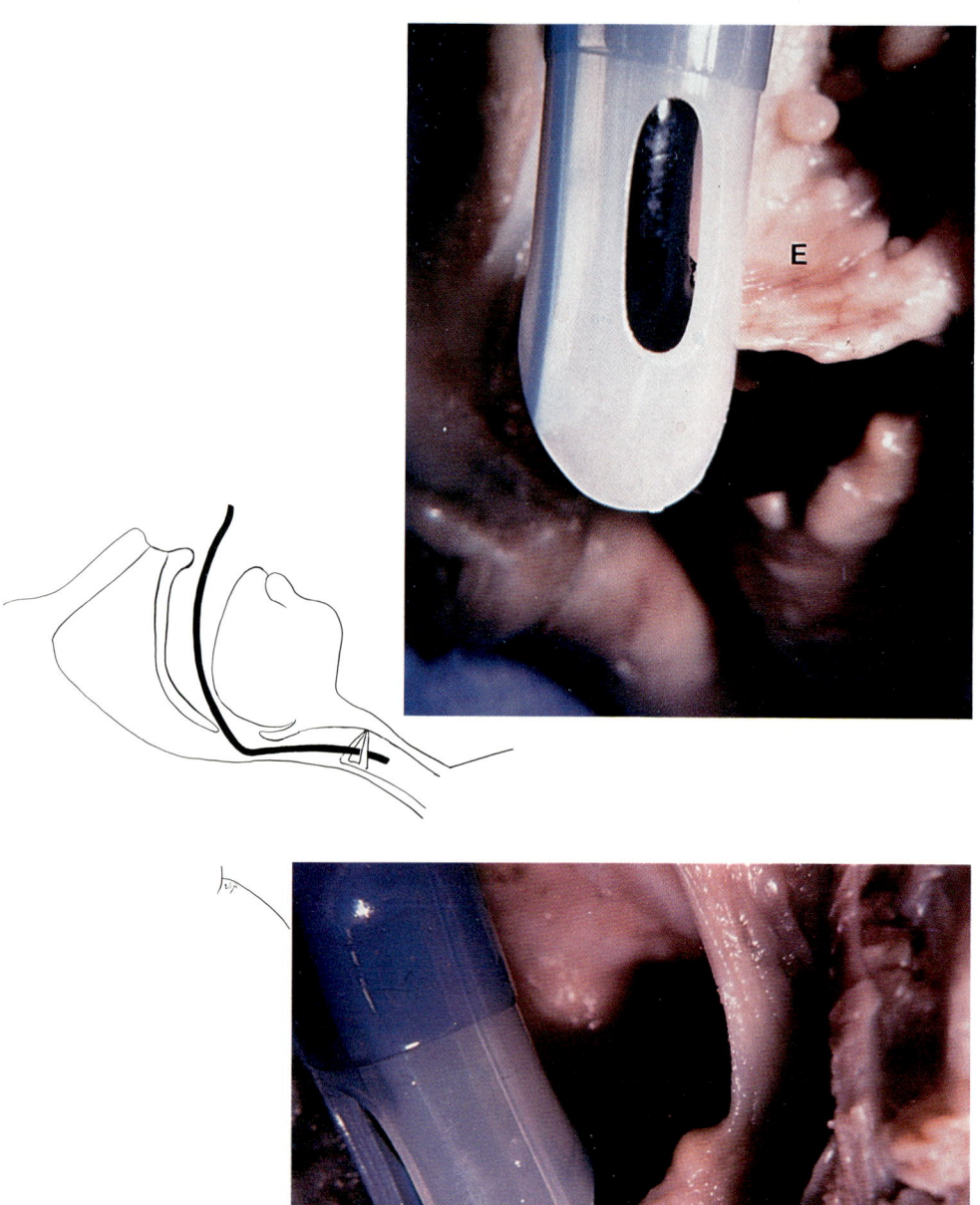

Fig 5–31.—During orotracheal intubation, the insertion tube forms an acute angle in the pharynx for the larynx to be visualized. Threading an orotracheal ETT over the endoscope may be difficult because the bevel of the ETT tends to catch at the epiglottis (E) or aryepiglottic folds (A).

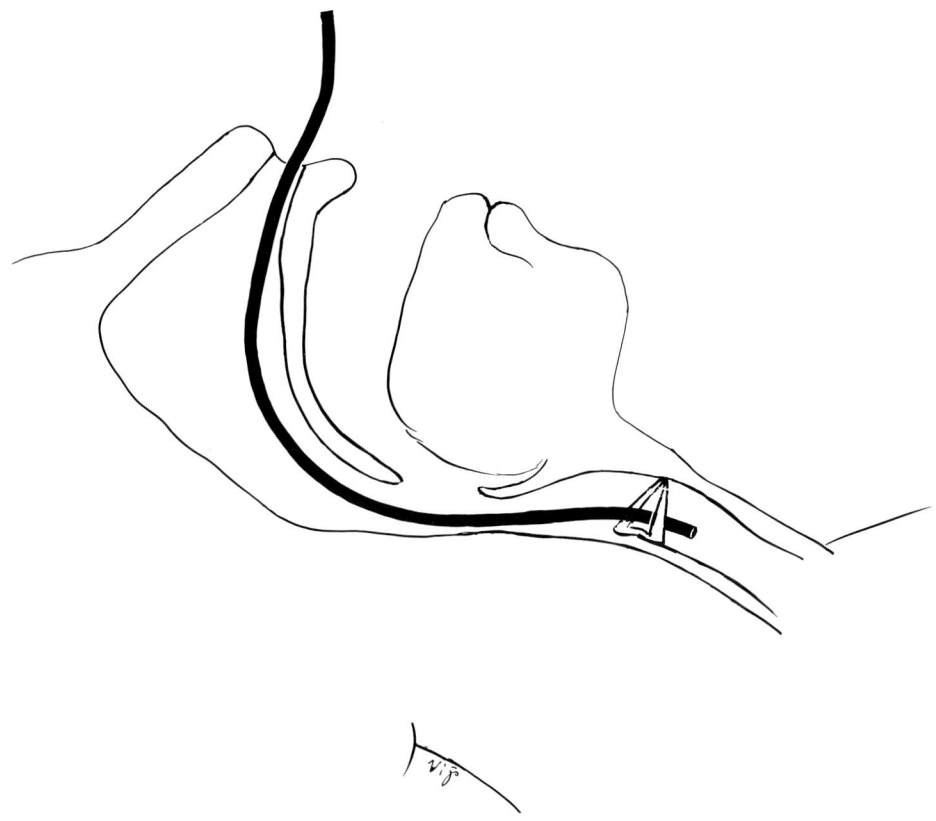

Fig 5–32.—It is relatively easier to visualize the larynx and thread the ETT during nasotracheal intubation because of the natural curve adopted by the insertion tube during its passage through the nasopharynx and pharynx.

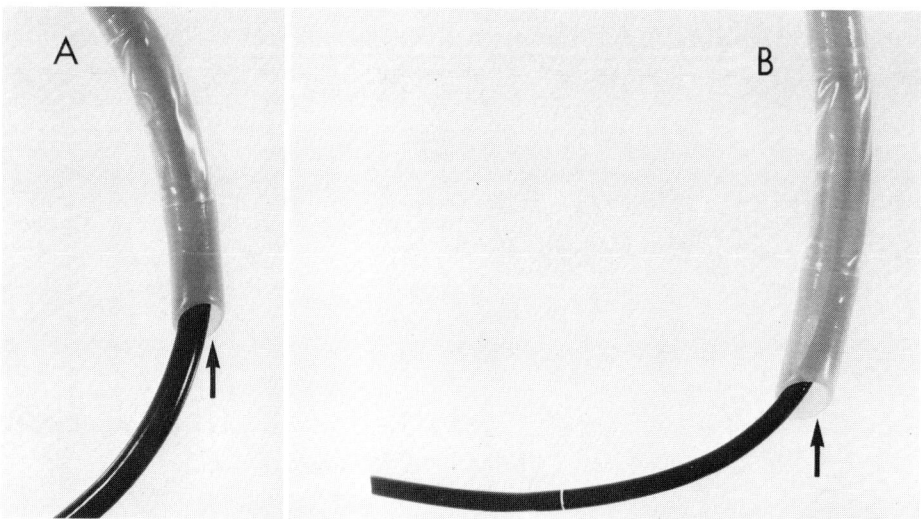

Fig 5–33.—It is easier to thread a large ETT over a large-diameter insertion tube **(A)** than one with a smaller diameter because the bevel of the ETT tends to impinge on the soft tissues and not follow the curve of the insertion tube **(B).**

USE OF AN INTUBATION GAUGE

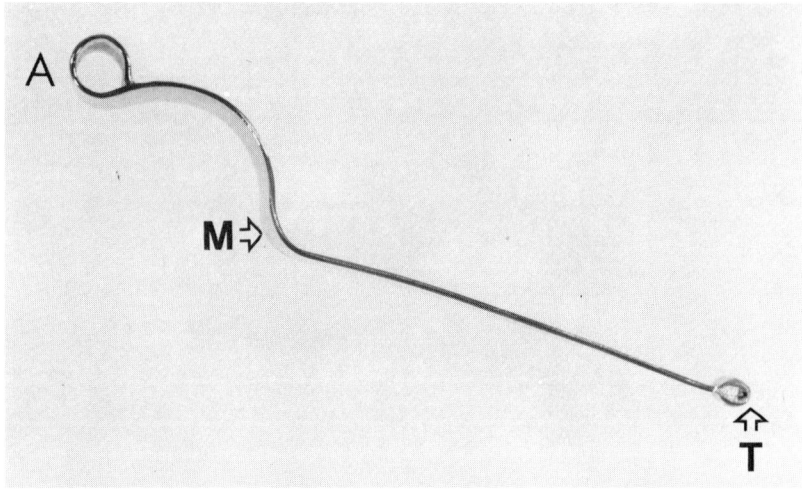

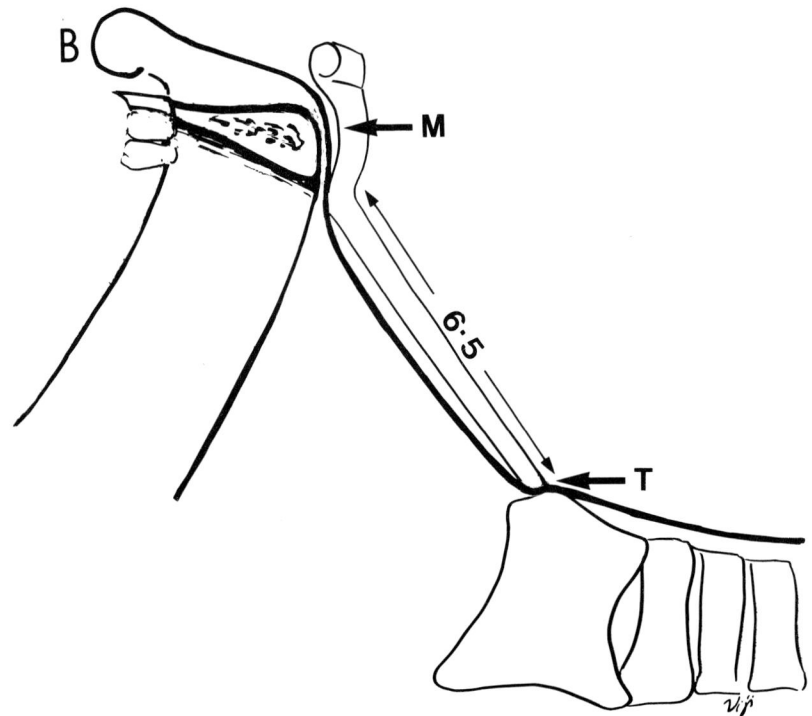

Fig 5–34.—An intubation gauge **(A)** can be used to estimate the degree of difficulty with endotracheal intubation. The distal end (T) is placed over the thyroid notch, and the angled part of the instrument (M) is placed under the lower border of the mandible. The length between T and M is 6.5 cm **(B)**.

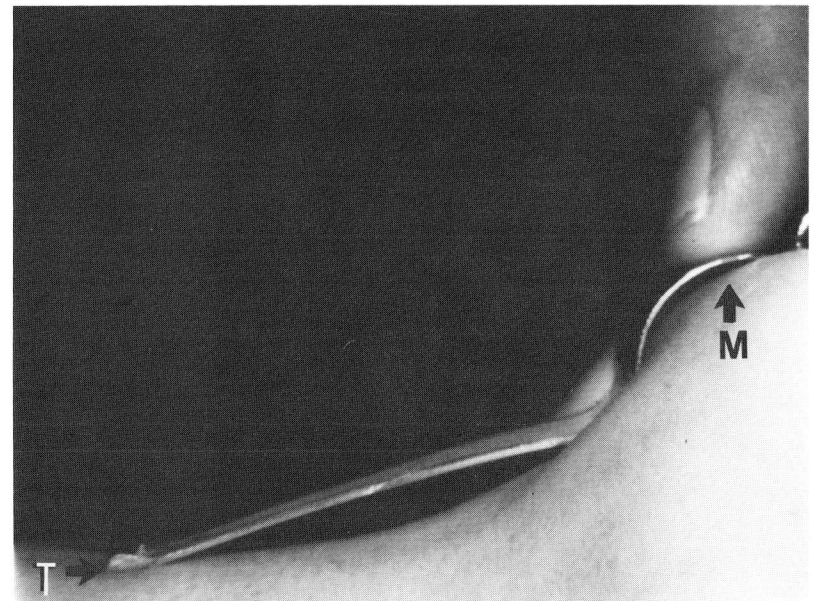

Fig 5–35.—In the normal person the distance between the lower border of the mandible (M) and the thyroid notch (T) is greater than 6.5 cm.

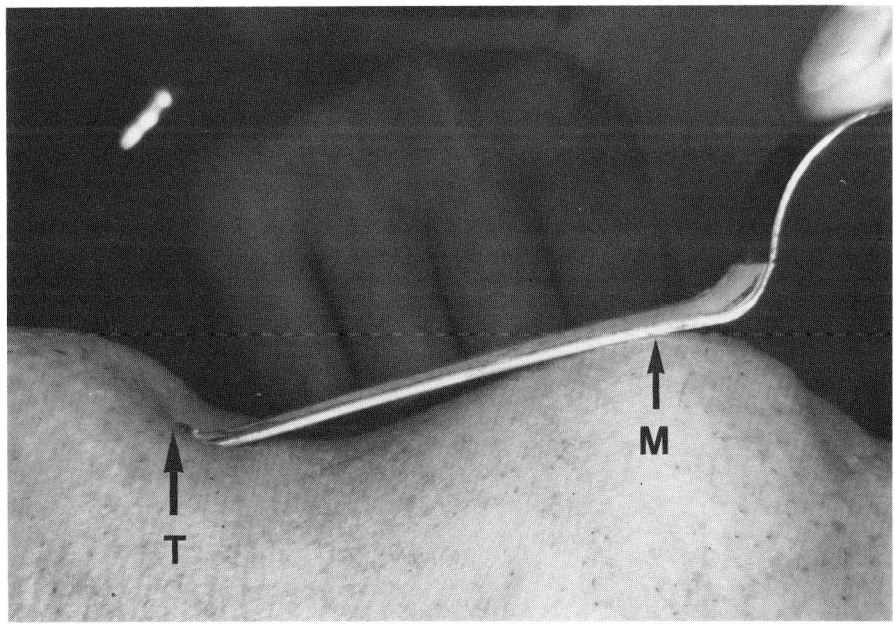

Fig 5–36.—When the distance is shorter than 6 cm, visualization of the larynx by direct laryngoscopy is impossible.

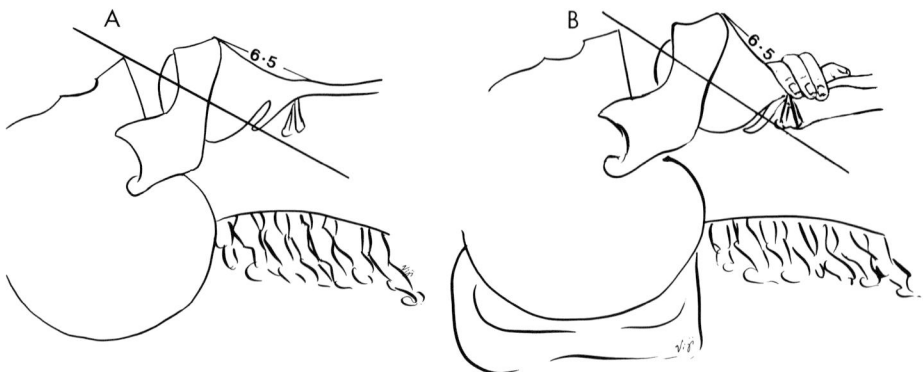

Fig 5–37.—When the distance between the lower border of the mandible and the thyroid notch is 6–6.5 cm, it can be predicted that the larynx will be visualized only with difficulty **(A)**. Direct laryngoscopy may be facilitated by using a straight blade, exerting pressure on the trachea, and placing a pillow under the head **(B)**.

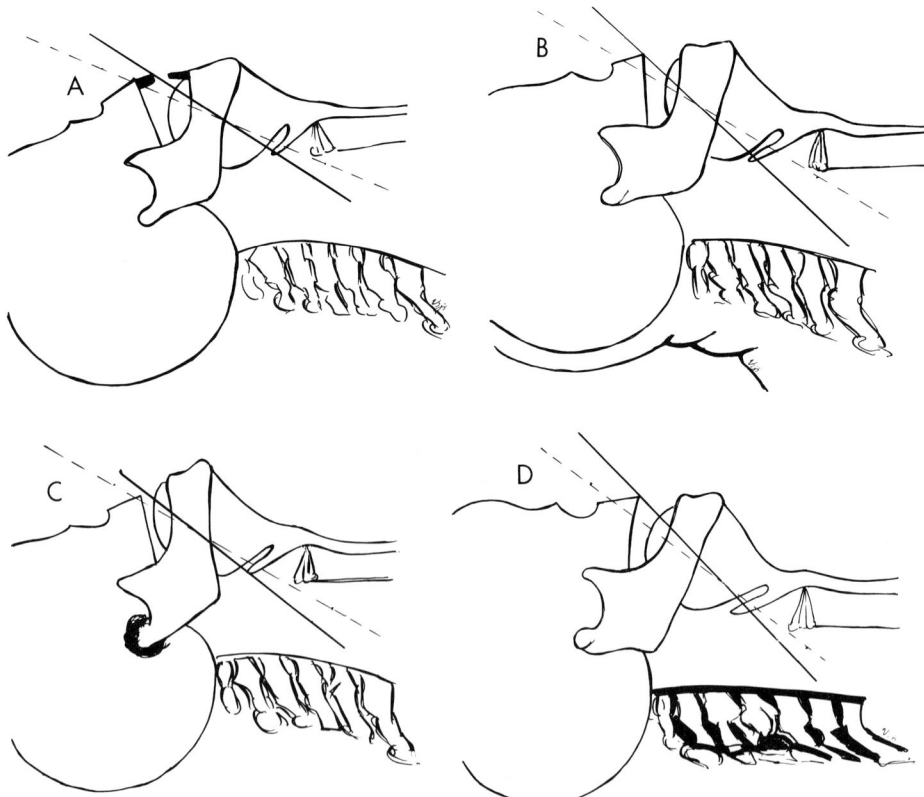

Fig 5–38.—When the distance between the thyroid notch and the lower border of the mandible is 6–6.5 cm and the patient has protruding teeth **(A)**, a thick neck **(B)**, temporomandibular joint ankylosis **(C)**, or ankylosis of the cervical spine **(D)**, visualization of the larynx by direct laryngoscopy usually is not possible. The *dashed lines* indicate the line of vision in the absence of these conditions.

ENDOSCOPIC INTUBATION IN CHILDREN

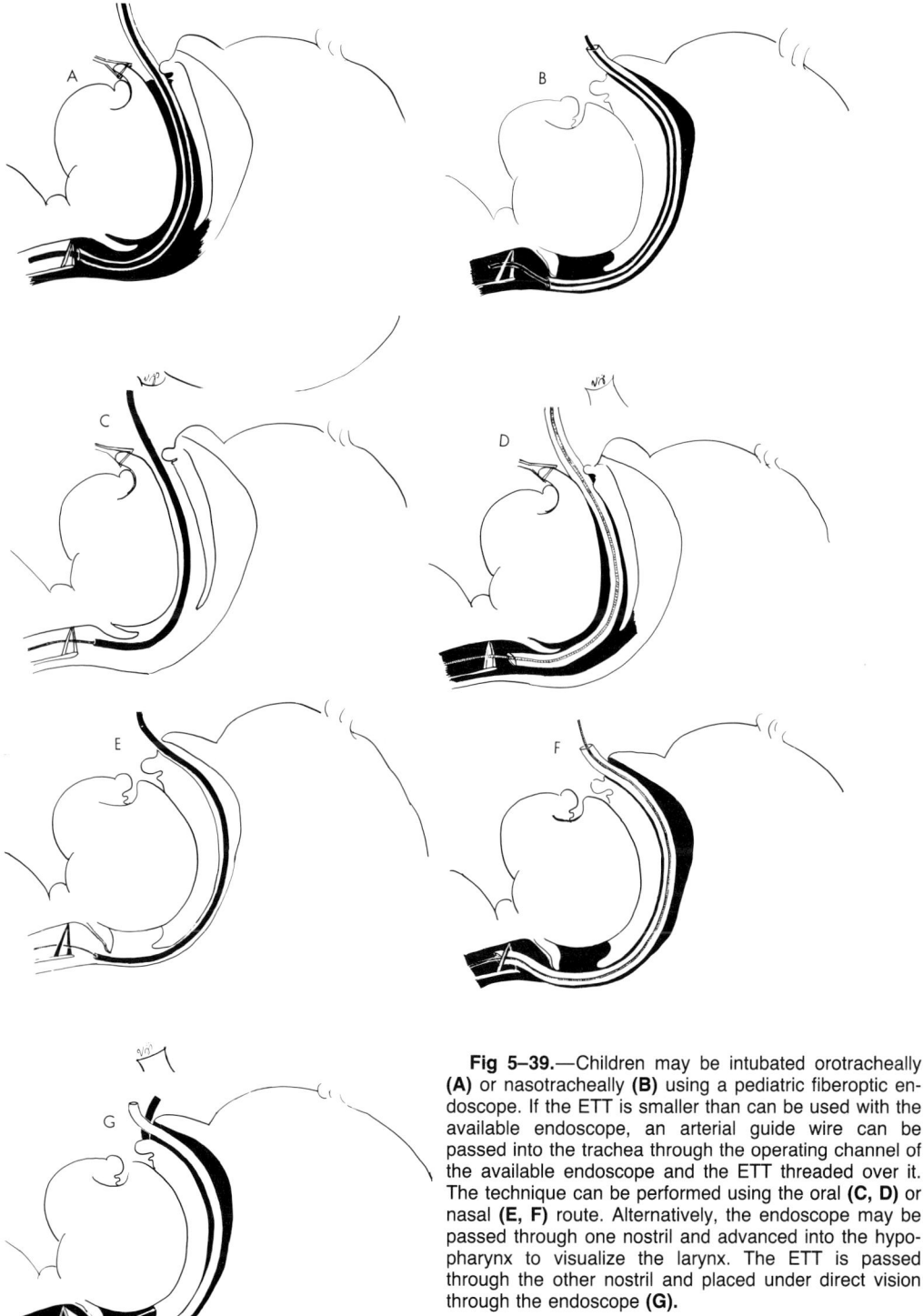

Fig 5–39.—Children may be intubated orotracheally **(A)** or nasotracheally **(B)** using a pediatric fiberoptic endoscope. If the ETT is smaller than can be used with the available endoscope, an arterial guide wire can be passed into the trachea through the operating channel of the available endoscope and the ETT threaded over it. The technique can be performed using the oral **(C, D)** or nasal **(E, F)** route. Alternatively, the endoscope may be passed through one nostril and advanced into the hypopharynx to visualize the larynx. The ETT is passed through the other nostril and placed under direct vision through the endoscope **(G)**.

6 / Clinical Applications

ALTHOUGH THE PRIMARY indication for fiberoptic laryngoscopy is endotracheal intubation of patients with abnormal airway anatomy, there are other diagnostic and therapeutic uses, including investigation of suspected airway pathology. Endotracheal tubes can be changed, their position verified, and tracheobronchial toilet can safely be performed in the operating room or intensive care unit with the aid of fiberoptic endoscopy (Table 6–1).

TABLE 6–1.—CLINICAL APPLICATIONS OF FIBEROPTIC ENDOSCOPY

Evaluation of airway pathology
  Congenital anomalies
  Trauma
  Tumor
  Inhalation injury
  Infection
  Nerve injury
  Difficult, traumatic, or prolonged intubation
Performance of endotracheal intubation in difficult situations
  Receding mandible, anterior larynx
  Obesity
  Rheumatoid arthritis
  Cervical spine fracture
  Temporomandibular joint ankylosis
  Distortion due to surgery, radiation, burns
Confirmation of tube placement
  Endotracheal
  Endobronchial
  Double lumen
  Tracheostomy
Positioning selective segmental blockers
Changing endotracheal tubes
Performing tracheobronchial toilet
Placement of nasogastric tubes

EVALUATION OF AIRWAY PATHOLOGY

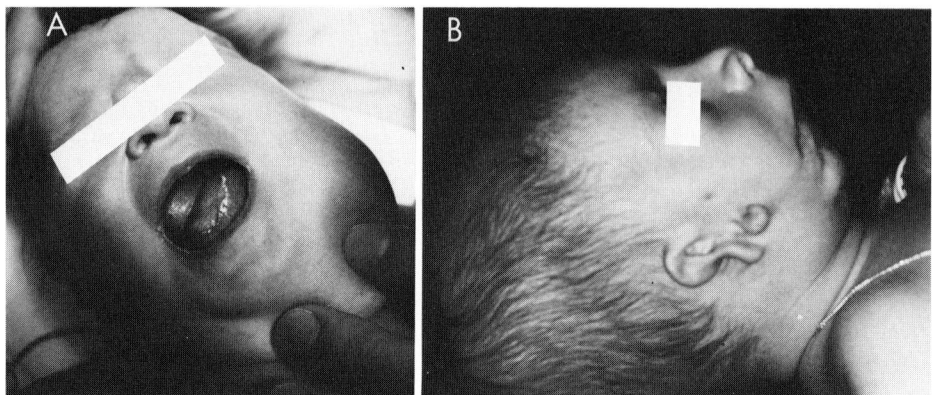

Fig 6–1.—Fiberoptic laryngoscopy can be used in children when difficulty with endotracheal intubation is anticipated. **A,** 6-month-old with cystic hygroma. **B,** 2-year-old with Goldenhar's syndrome.

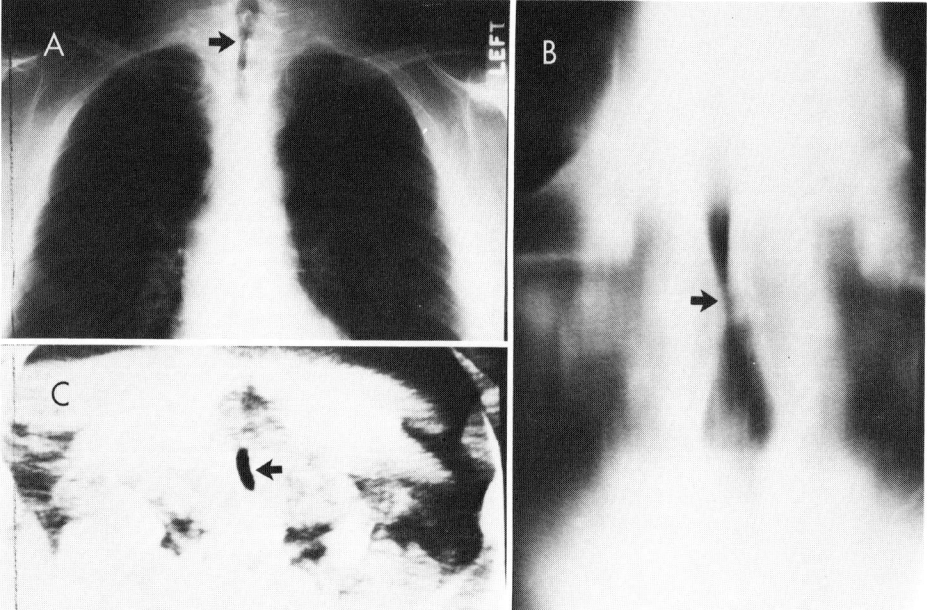

Fig 6–2.—Tumors may produce extrinsic compression of the airway. Chest x-ray **(A)** and tomogram **(B)** of the neck demonstrating narrowing of the trachea. CT scan **(C)** confirming that lateral pressure is due to an enlarged thyroid gland. Endoscopic appearance of trachea prior to endotracheal intubation **(D).**

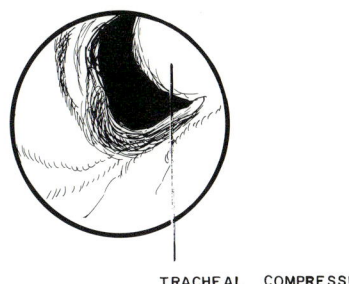
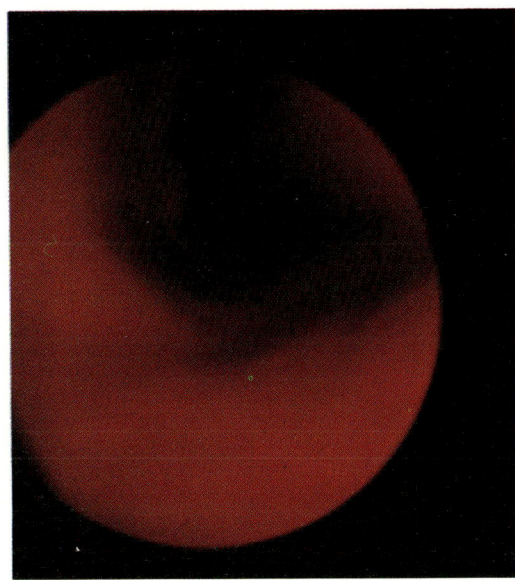

Fig 6–2 D.

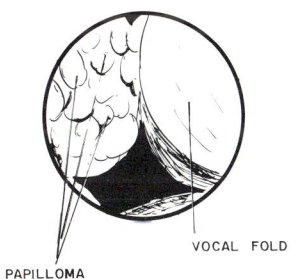
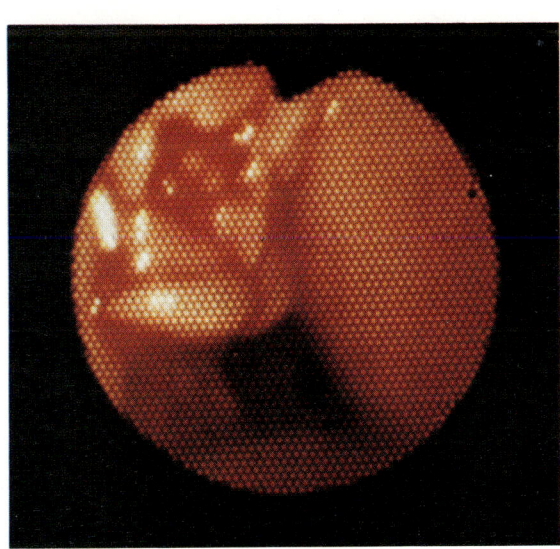

Fig 6–3.—Larynx of patient with recurrent respiratory papillomatosis.

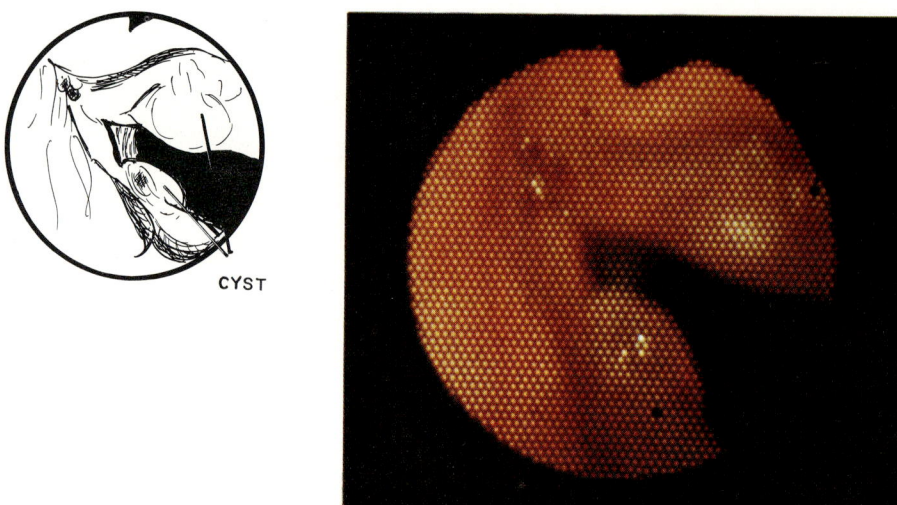

Fig 6–4.—Bilateral cystic lesions of the vocal folds.

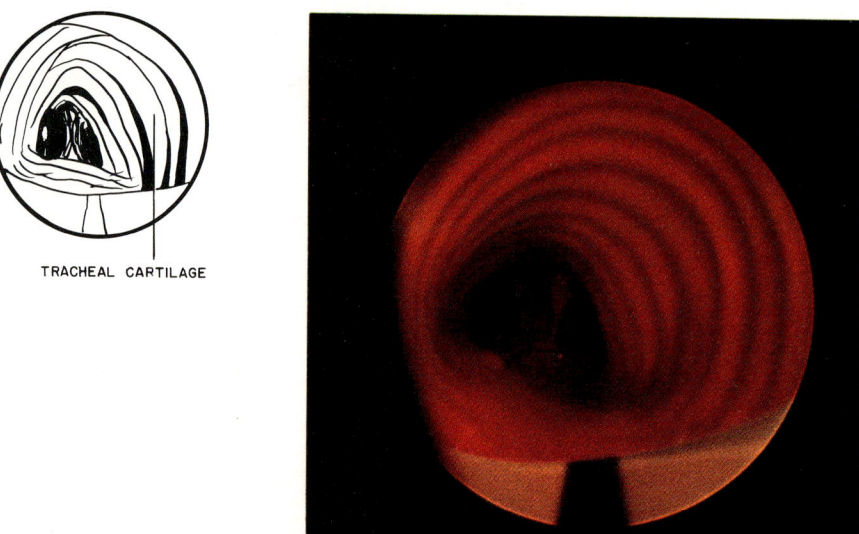

Fig 6–5.—Erythematous trachea following inhalation injury.

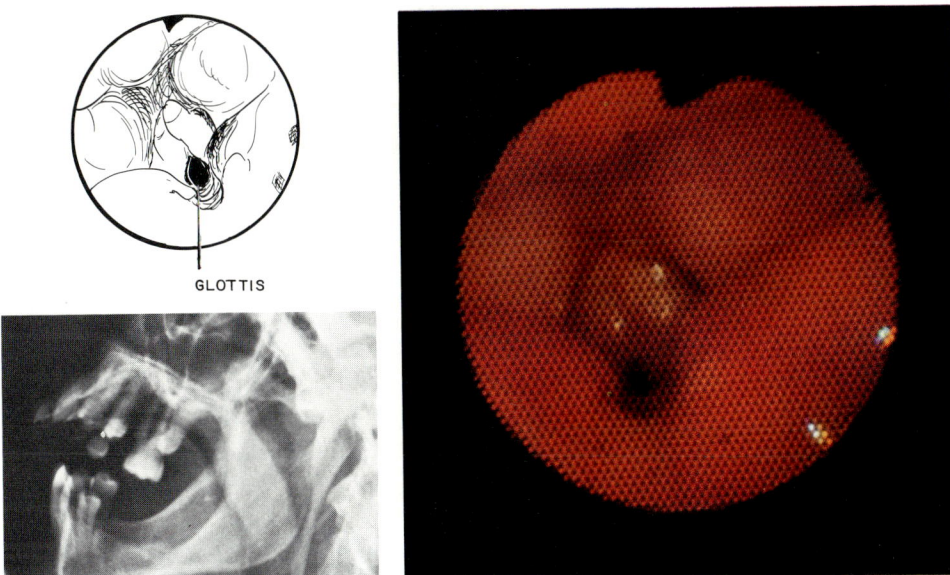

Fig 6–6.—Inflammatory reaction of the aryepiglottic and vestibular folds virtually obscuring the glottis in a patient who had prominent upper teeth and limited range of motion of the temporomandibular joint, which precluded direct laryngoscopy.

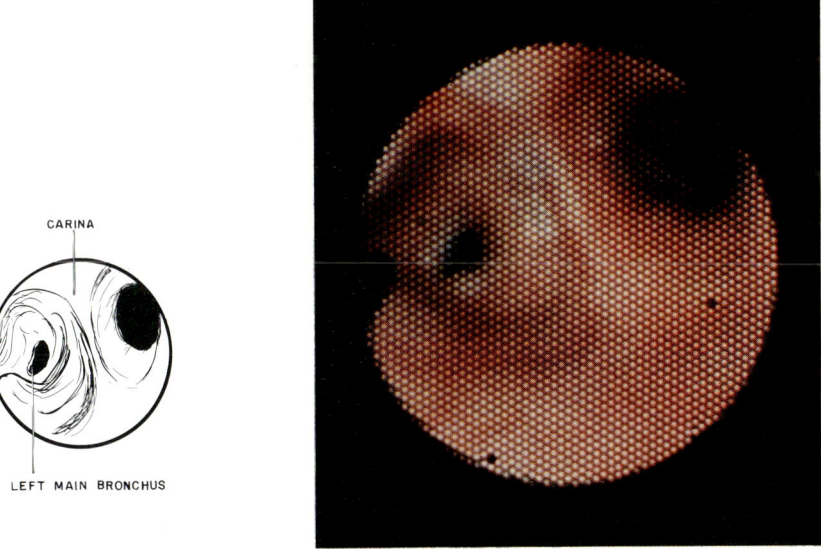

Fig 6–7.—Narrowing and straightening of the left main bronchus in a patient with chronic bronchitis.

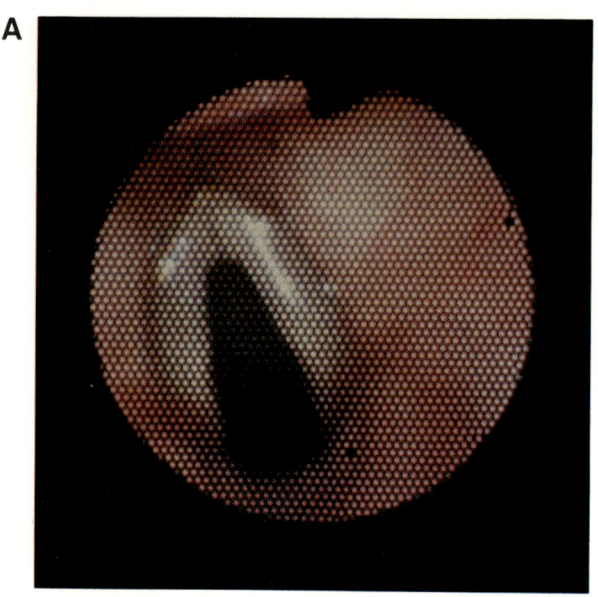

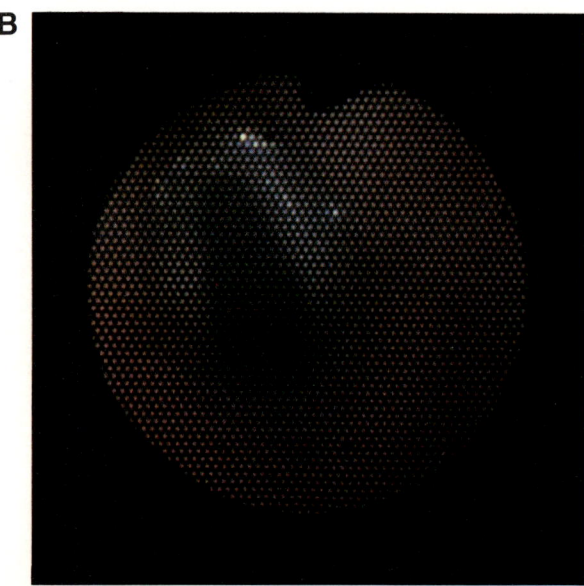

Fig 6–8.—Following surgical procedures in which damage to the recurrent laryngeal nerves may occur, fiberoptic laryngoscopy may be used to evaluate movement of the vocal folds. Even in normal persons, there is little change in the aperture of the glottis during inspiration **(A)** and expiration **(B)** during spontaneous breathing. Fogging of the lens occurs during expiration.

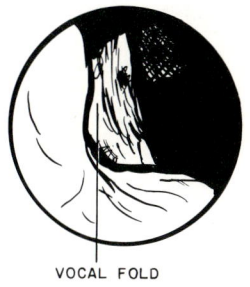
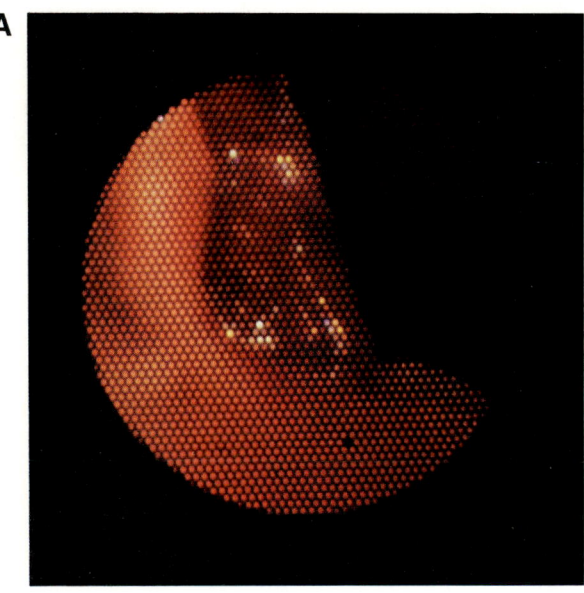
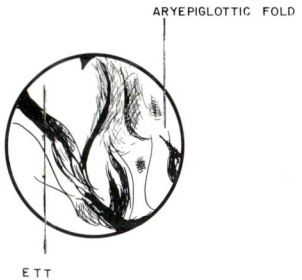
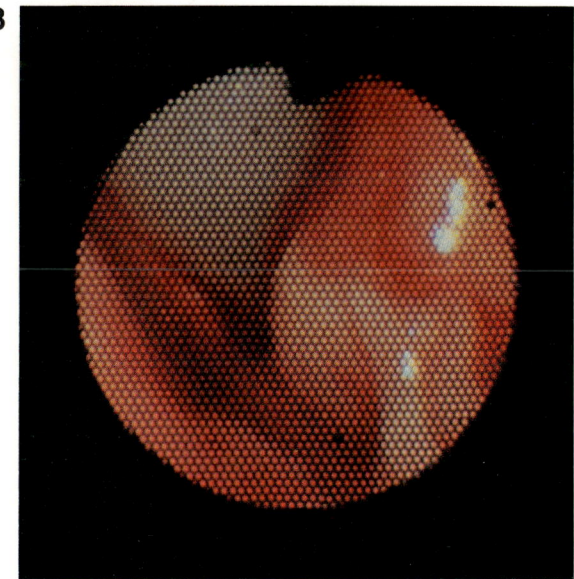

Fig 6–9.—Hemorrhage **(A)** and edema **(B)** resulting from traumatic endotracheal intubation.

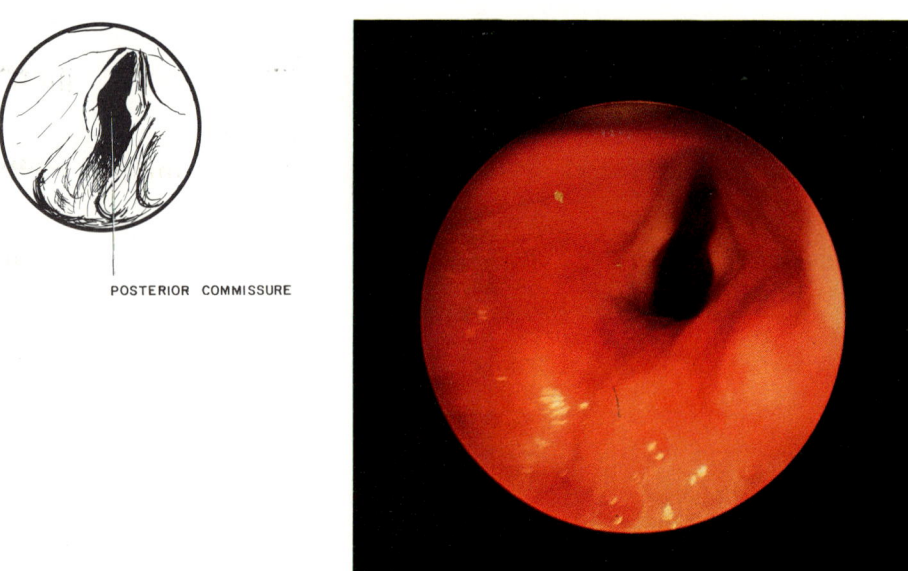

Fig 6–10.—Appearance of the larynx one week following extubation in a patient who had been intubated for three weeks. The depressed area extending from the posterior commissure to the corniculate cartilages and the irregular vocal folds resulted from prolonged contact with the ETT.

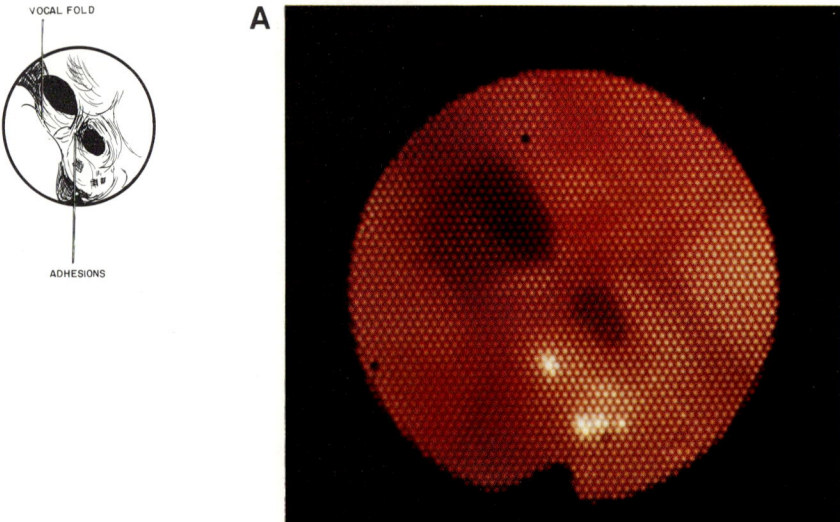

Fig 6–11.—Fibrous band between the vocal folds **(A)** and in the trachea **(B)** following prolonged endotracheal intubation.

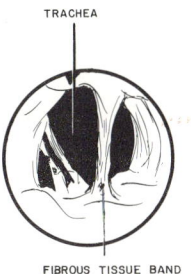
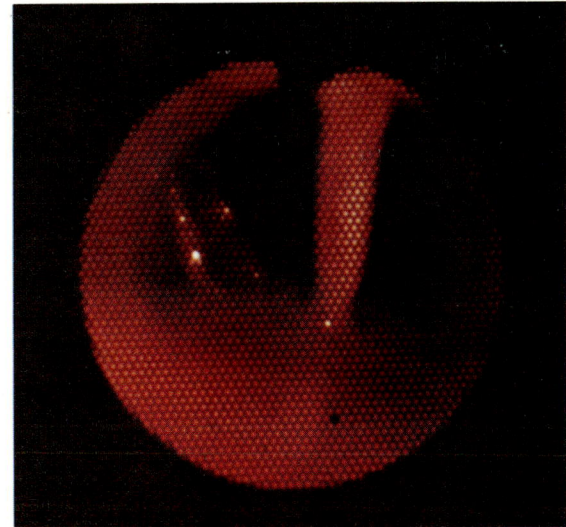

Fig 6–11 B.

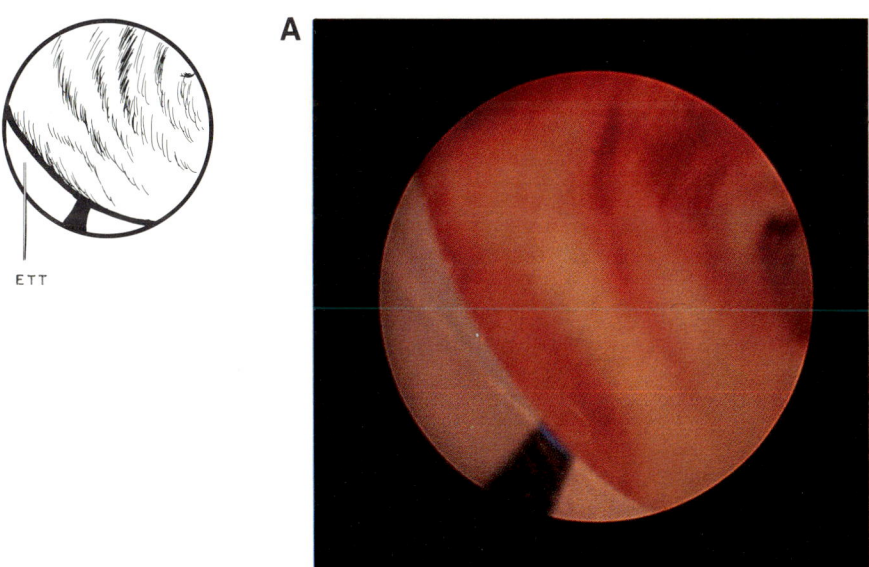

Fig 6–12.—**A,** blanched area in trachea following prolonged contact with inflated ETT cuff. Hemorrhagic area **(B)** distal to the end of the ETT.

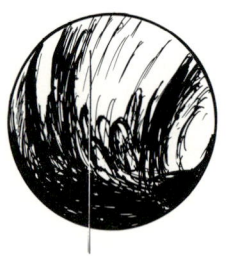

TRACHEAL CARTILAGE

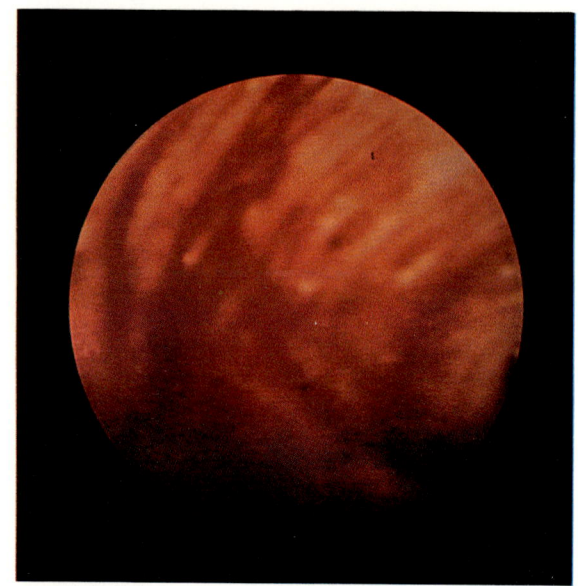

Fig 6–12 B.

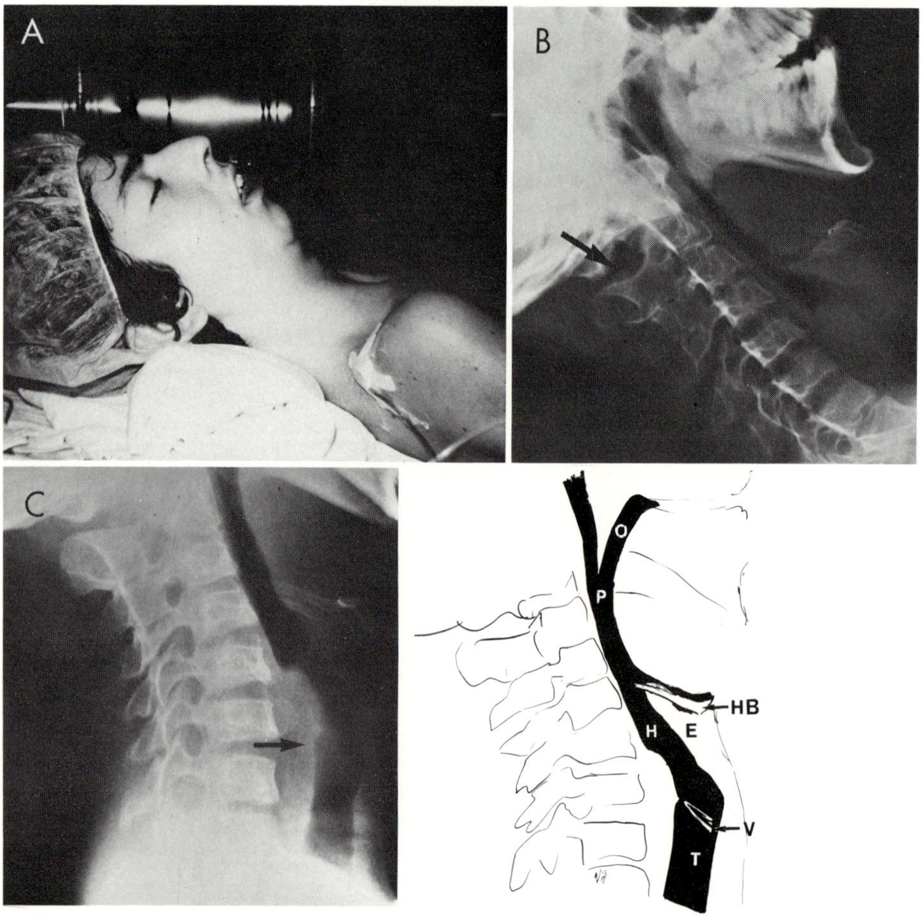

Fig 6–13.—A, receding mandible in patient with severe juvenile rheumatoid arthritis. **B,** x-ray of cervical spine taken in maximum possible extension demonstrates complete ankylosis. **C,** larynx is extremely anterior. O = oropharynx, P = pharynx, H = hypopharynx, HB = hyoid bone, E = epiglottis, V = vocal folds, T = trachea.

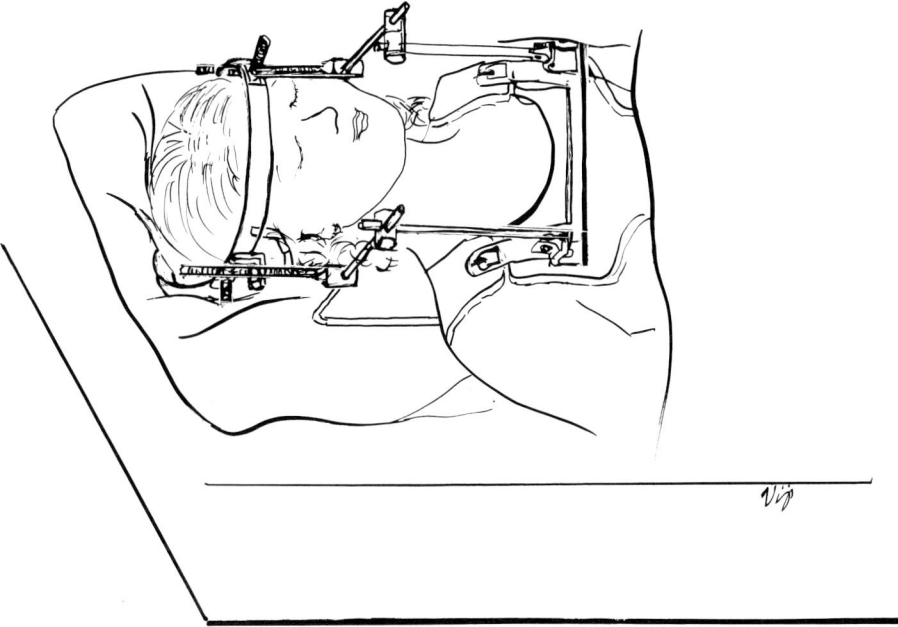

Fig 6–14.—The presence of Halo traction severely limits movement of the neck. In many patients any manipulation of the cervical spine is contraindicated.

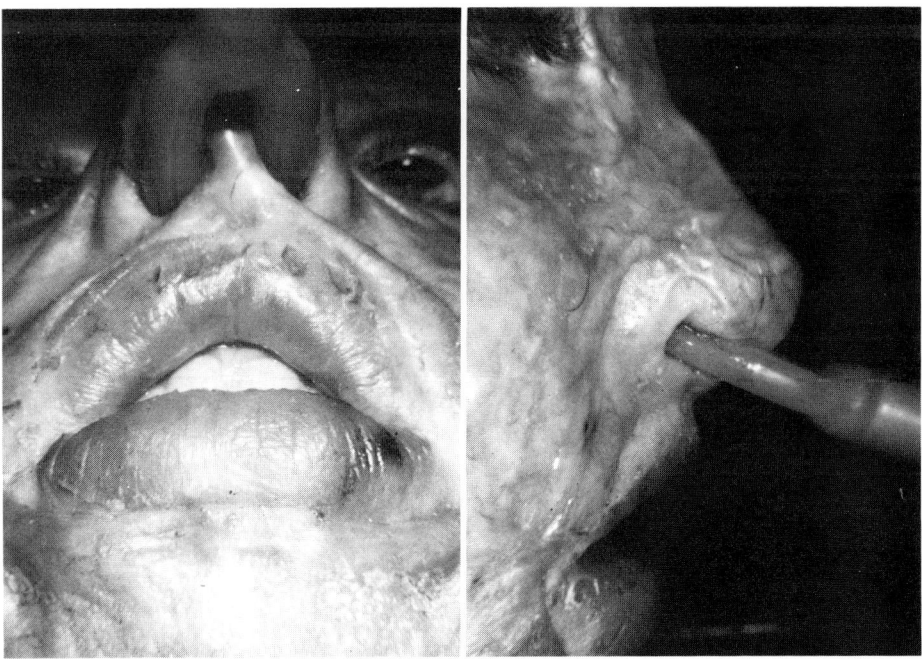

Fig 6–15.—Distortion of the mouth and nose due to scar contractures resulting from third-degree burn, making direct laryngoscopy impossible.

CONFIRMATION OF TUBE PLACEMENT

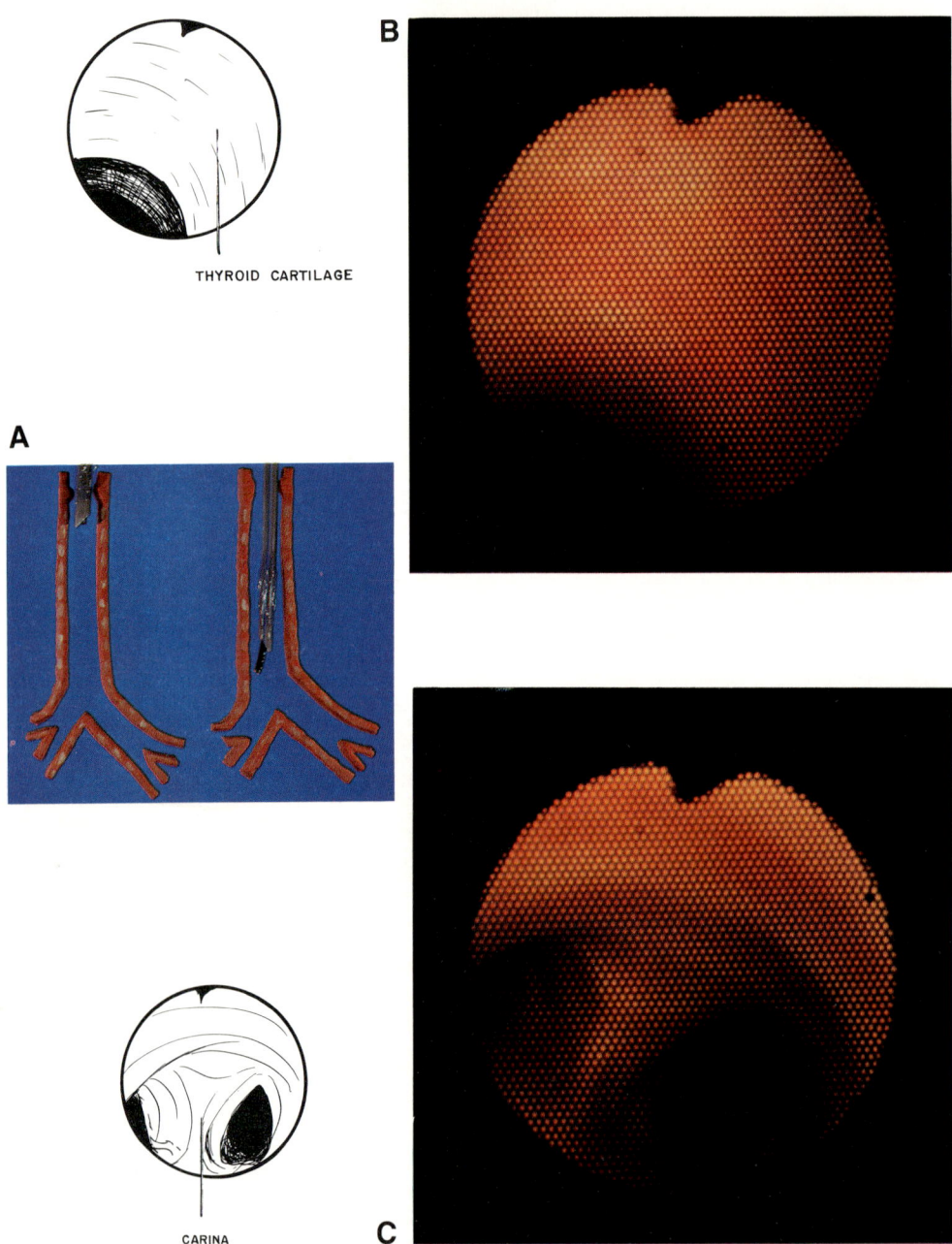

Fig 6–16.—Fiberoptic endoscopy is useful in confirming the position of ETTs. The insertion tube is threaded through the diaphragm of an endoscopic adapter, which permits ventilation during endoscopy and manipulation of the ETT. However, the presence of a relatively large insertion tube increases the resistance to gas flow. **A,** cuff of ETT above the vocal cords and properly positioned. Endoscopic view before **(B)** and after **(C)** repositioning of ETT.

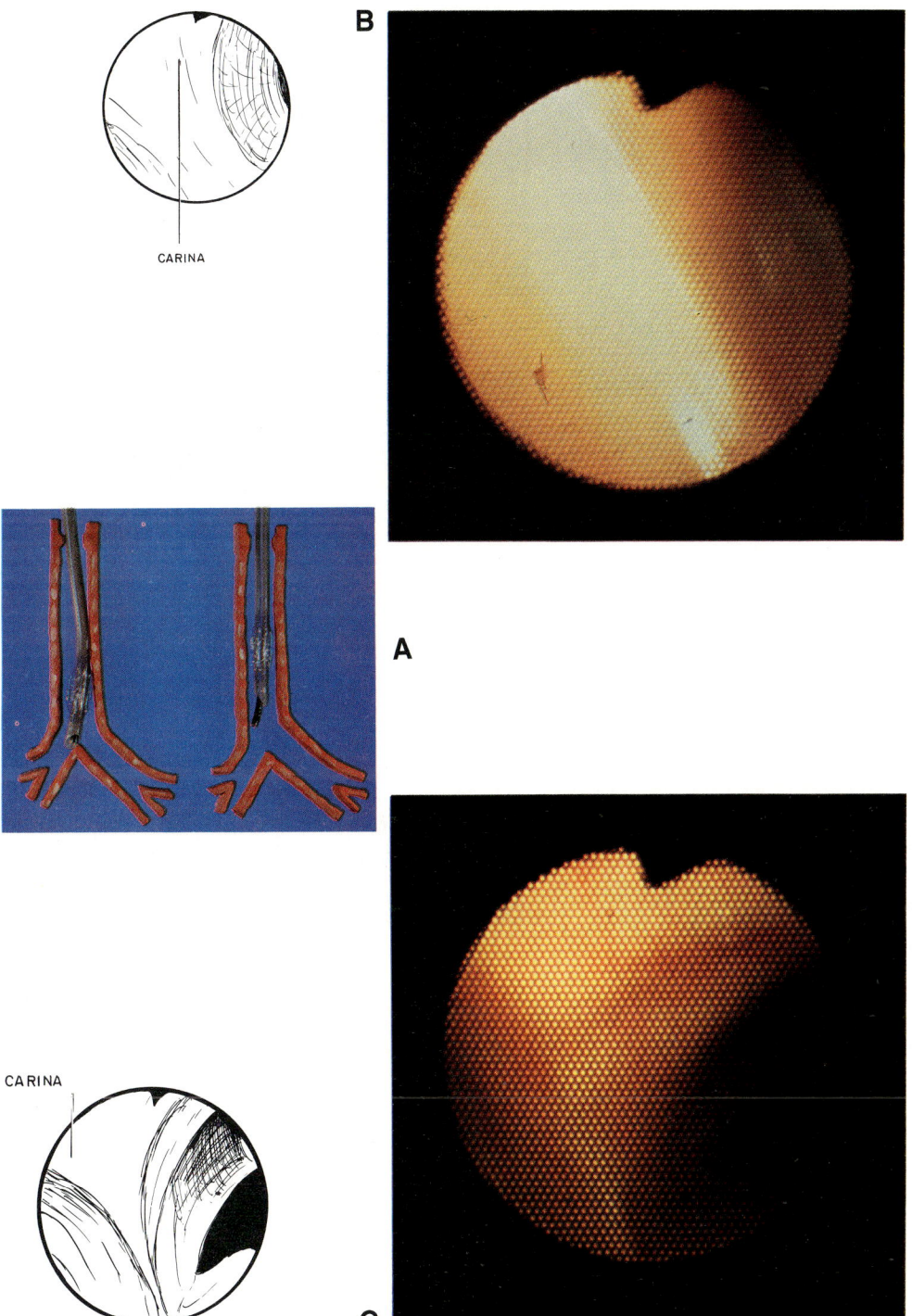

Fig 6–17.—A, ETT touching the carina and following repositioning in the trachea. When the insertion tube of the endoscope is very close to the carina, only light reflected from the carinal mucosa is seen. Endoscopic view before **(B)** and after **(C)** repositioning of the tube.

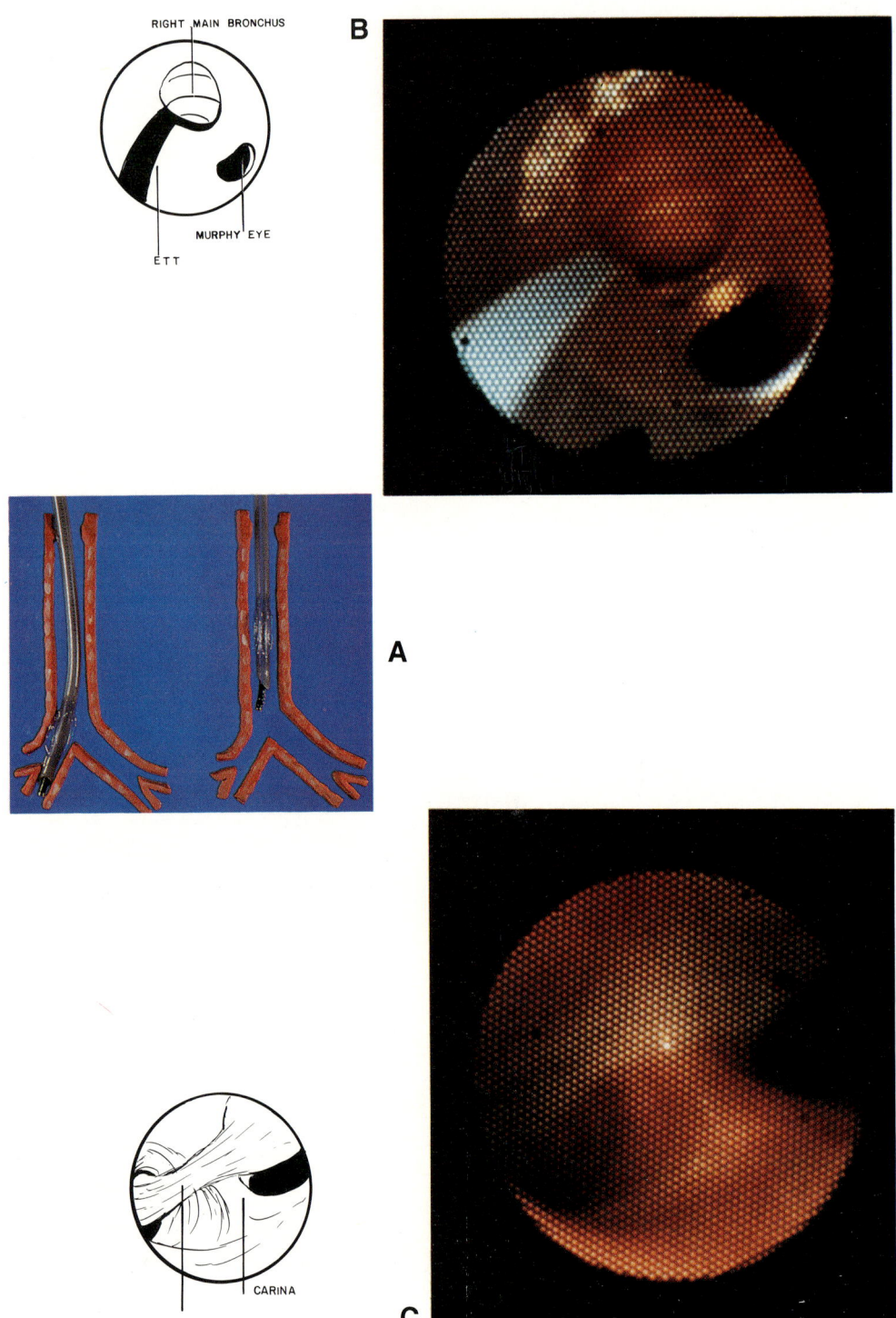

Fig 6–18.—**A,** ETT in the right main bronchus and properly positioned in the trachea. Endoscopic view before **(B)** and after **(C)** repositioning of the tube.

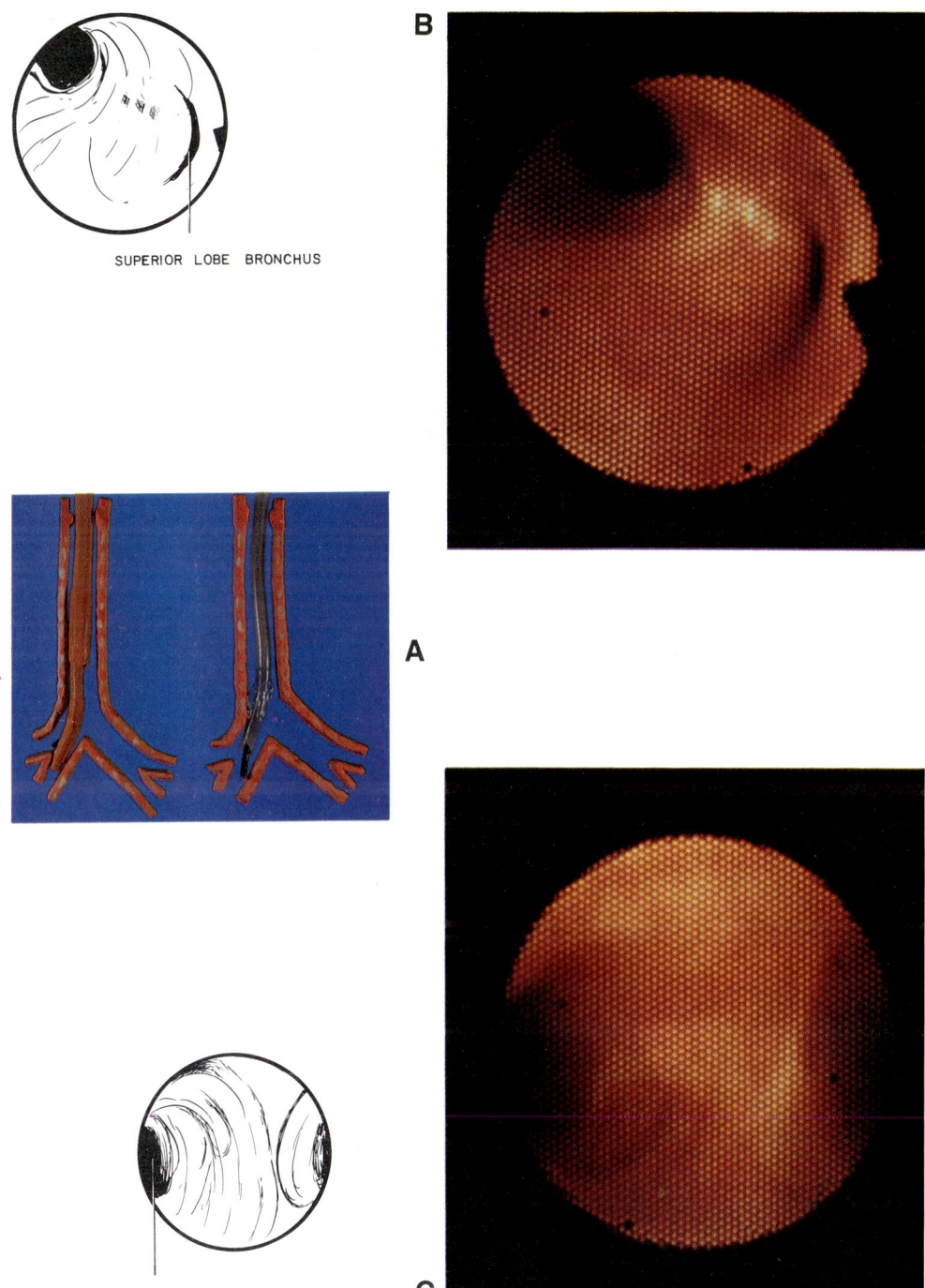

Fig 6–19.—A pediatric endoscope is used to position double-lumen and endobronchial tubes. **A,** the insertion tube is placed through the eye of the double-lumen tube or through the tip of the endobronchial tube to ascertain that the superior lobe bronchus is not occluded **(B).** Endoscopic view of the superior lobe bronchus **(C).** Endoscopic view of left main bronchus. Endoscopy can be repeated to reconfirm placement of the tube during the operative procedure.

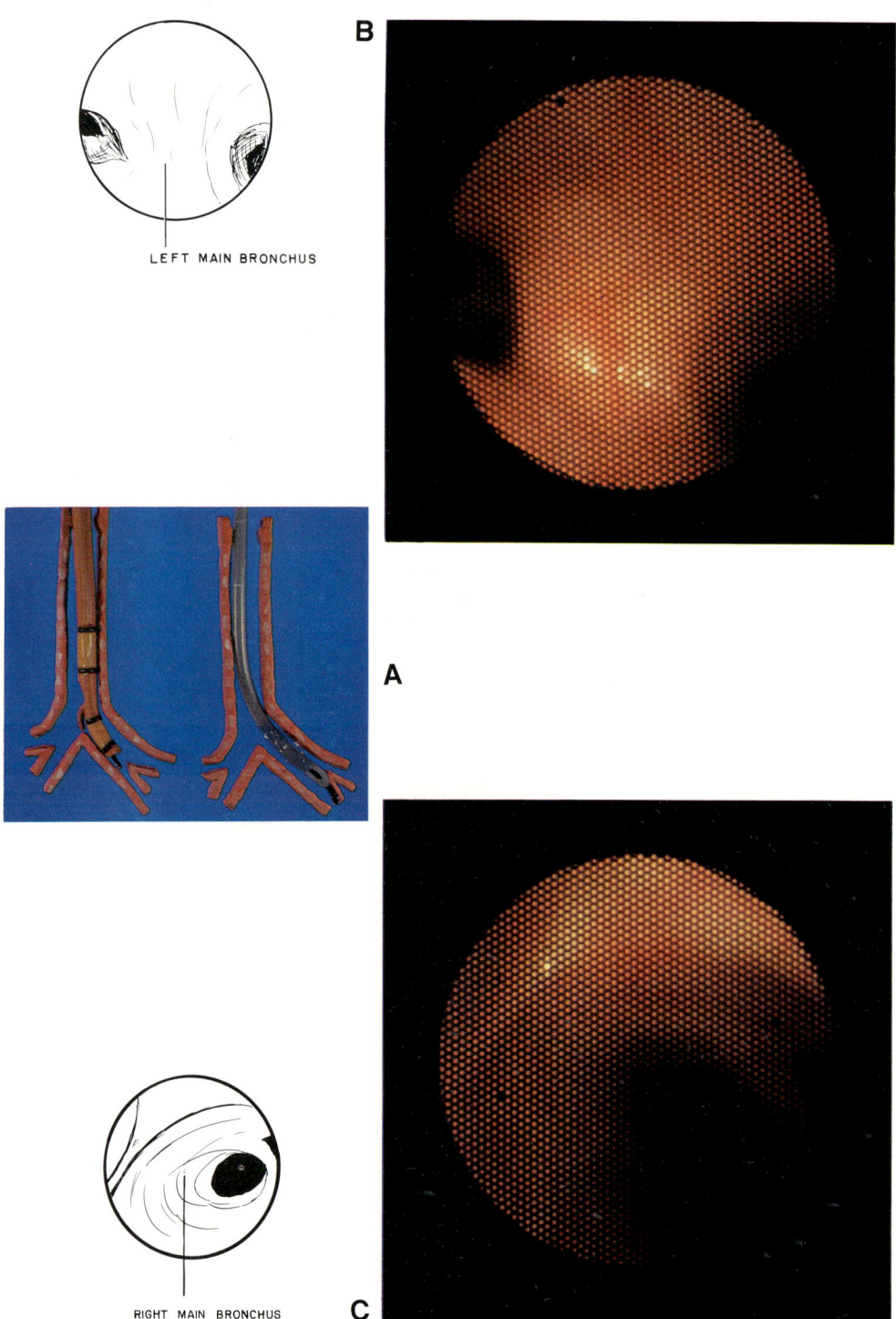

Fig 6–20.—A, Use of a pediatric endoscope to position a double-lumen tube or endobronchial tube in the left main bronchus **(B).** Endoscopic view of the left main bronchus **(C).** Endoscopic view of the right main bronchus.

POSITIONING SEGMENTAL BRONCHIAL BLOCKERS

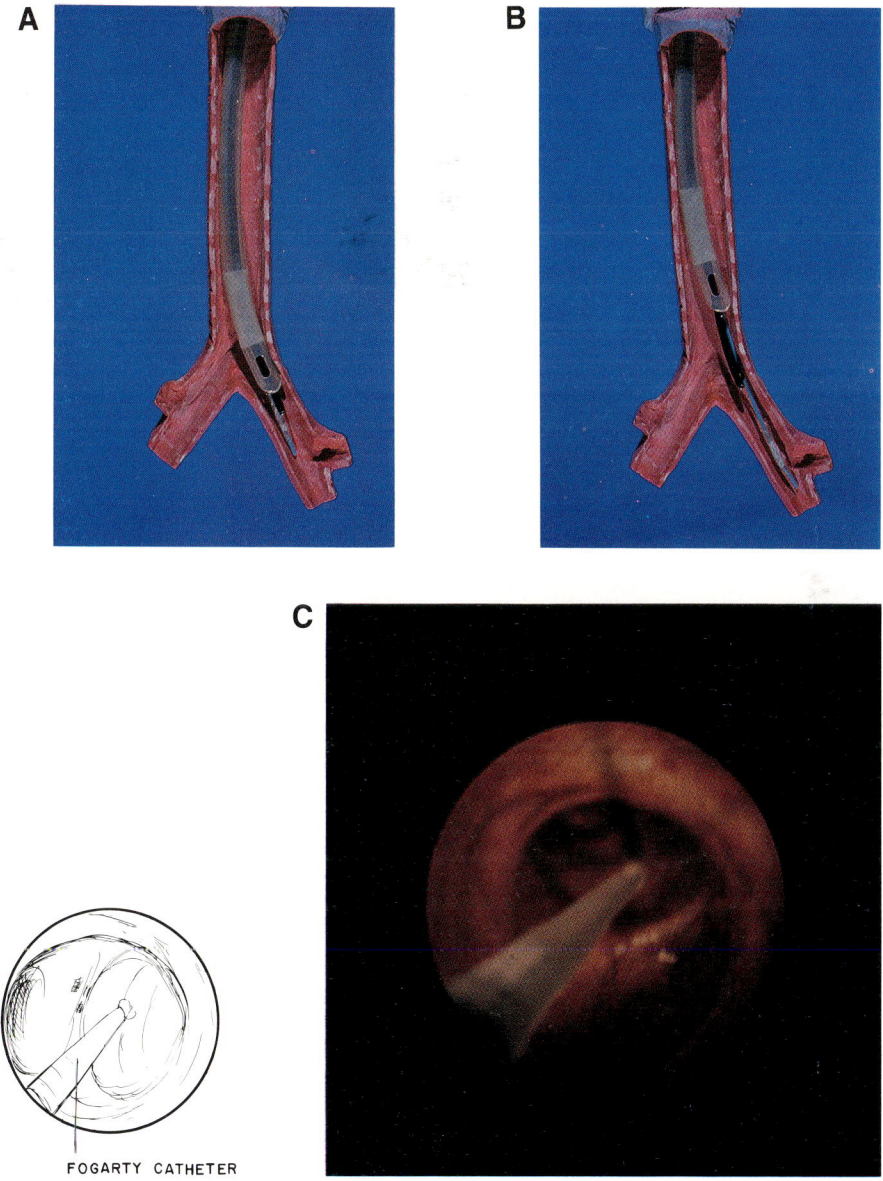

Fig 6–21.—A pediatric endoscope can be used to selectively place a bronchial blocker. The ETT is advanced into the desired bronchus using the endoscope. **A,** Fogarty catheter is placed beside the insertion tube and **(B)** threaded into the bronchus **(C).** The catheter is in the segment to be blocked.

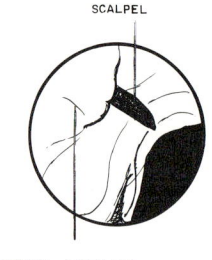
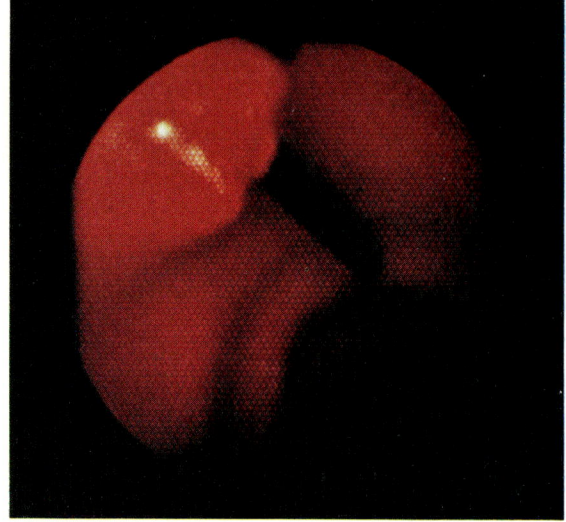

A

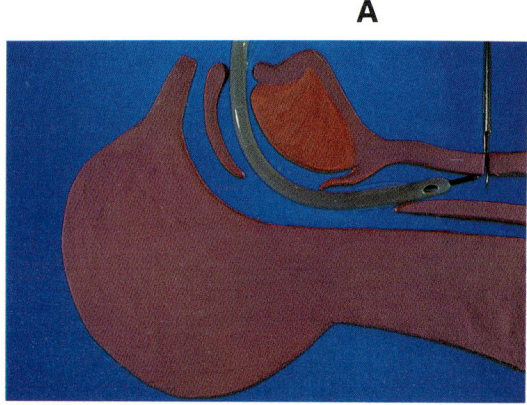

Fig 6–22.—Most tracheostomies are performed with an ETT in situ. The ETT is withdrawn above the level of the tracheal incision prior to insertion of the tracheostomy tube. A fiberoptic endoscope can be placed within the ETT to visualize the intratracheal portion of the operation and to ascertain proper placement of an appropriately sized tracheostomy tube. Use of this technique is especially valuable when: (1) endotracheal intubation was difficult, contraindicating removal of the ETT until proper placement of the tracheostomy is certain; (2) there is technical difficulty during the surgical procedure necessitating reinsertion of the ETT; and (3) there is question of the tracheostomy tube's being placed in a false passage. The ETT is withdrawn under direct vision above the level of the tracheal incision. The scalpel blade **(A)** and tracheostomy tube **(B)** are seen entering the tracheal lumen.

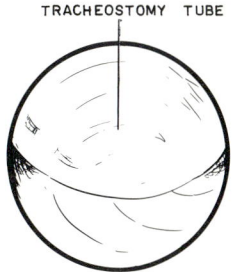
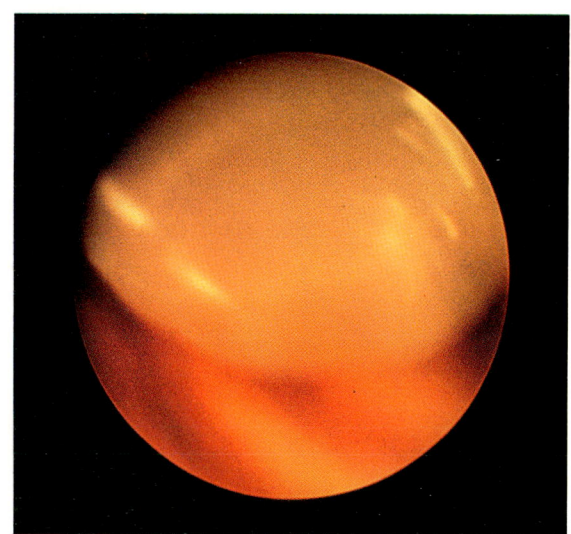
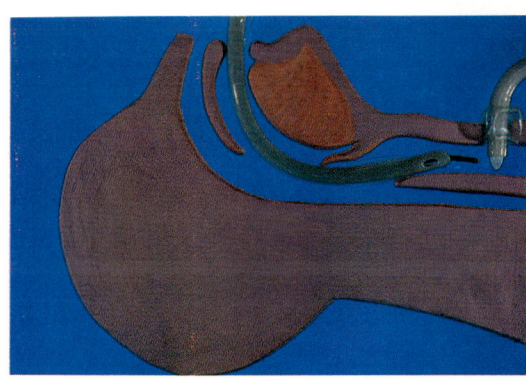

Fig 6–22 B.

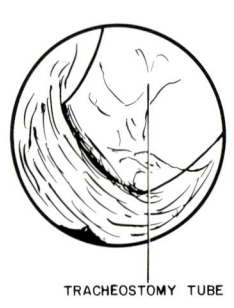

TRACHEOSTOMY TUBE

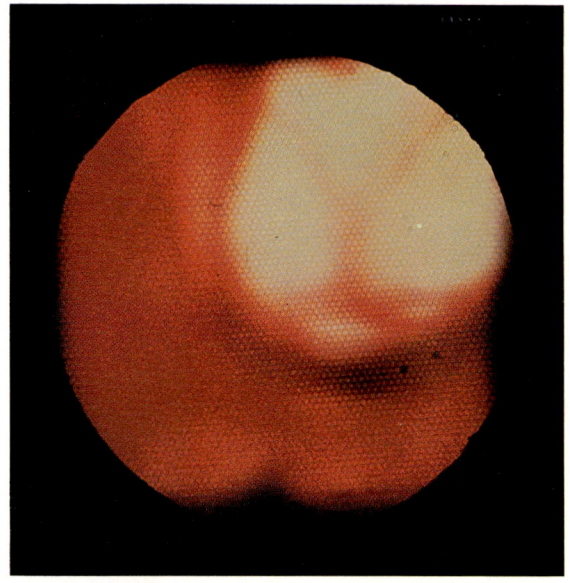

C

D

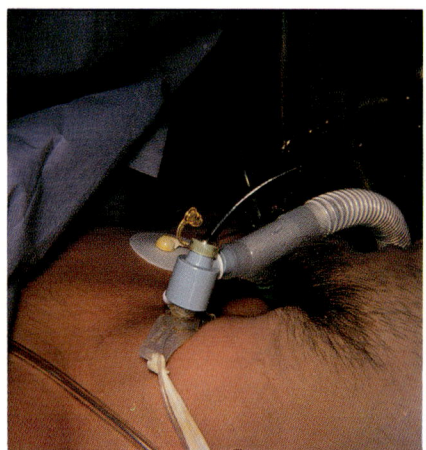

Fig 6–22. (cont.)—Proper placement of the tracheostomy tube is confirmed **(C)**. Endoscopy may be performed through the tracheostomy tube to assess the position of the tube relative to the carina **(D)**.

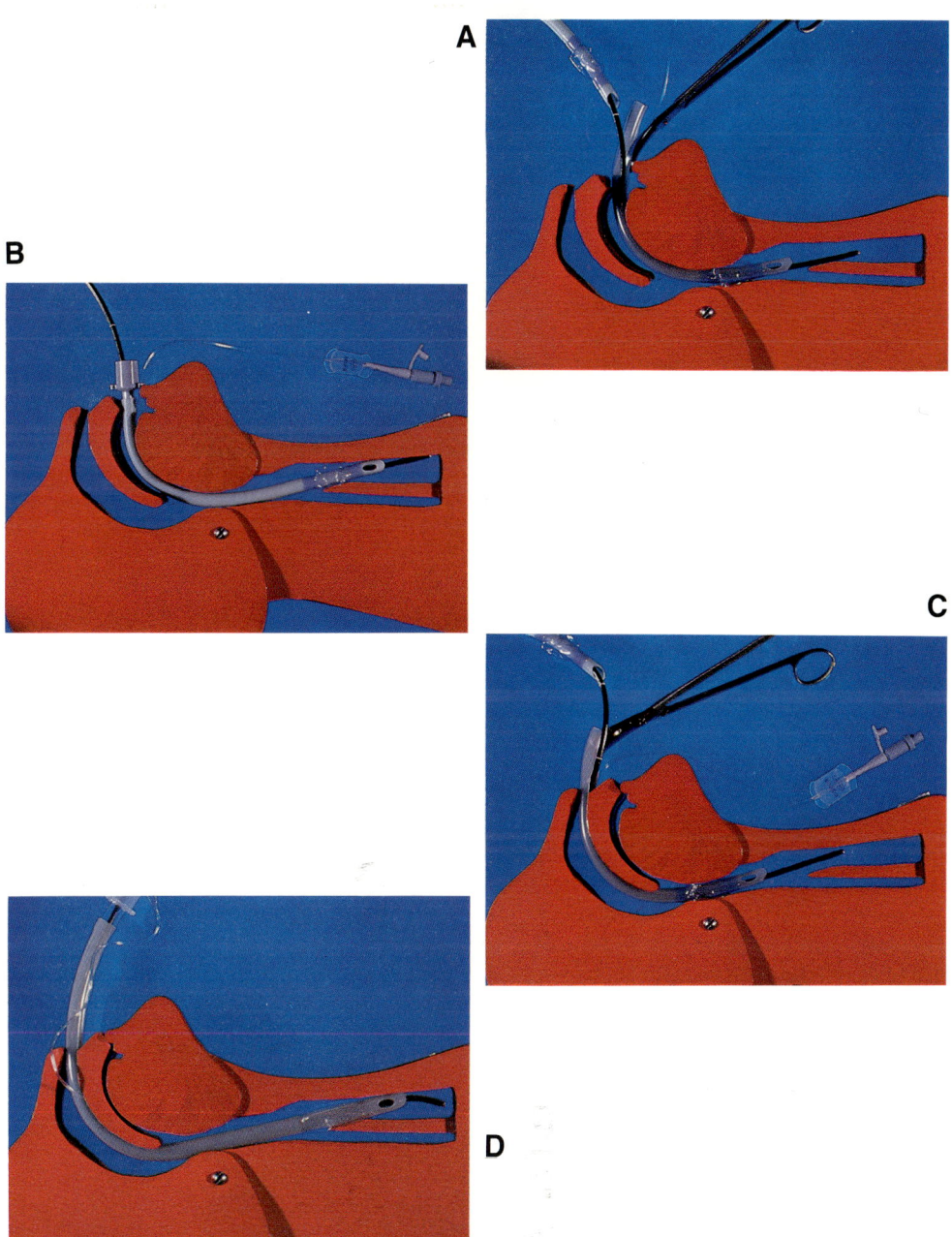

Fig 6–23.—Fiberoptic endoscopy facilitates changing ETTs. The technique allows insufflation of oxygen through the existing tube during the procedure; it is especially useful in patients in whom initial endotracheal intubation was difficult. The existing tube is slit longitudinally and withdrawn as the new ETT is advanced over the insertion tube of the endoscope. The new ETT may be placed either orotracheally **(A, B)** or nasotracheally **(C, D).**

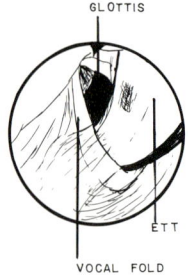
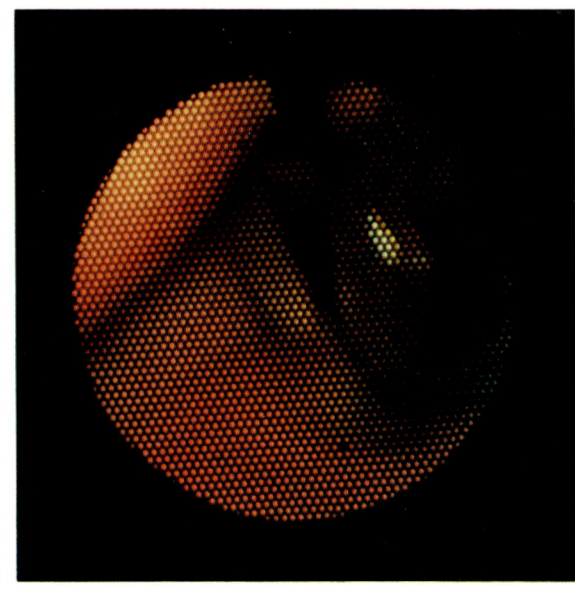

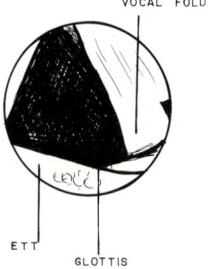
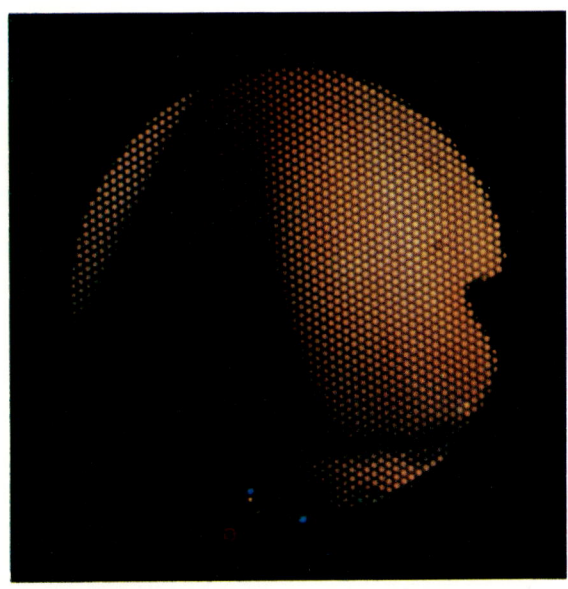

Fig 6–24.—An ETT normally lies in the posterior commissure rather than the anterior commissure **(A, B)**. When there is sufficient space, the insertion tube can be placed anterior to the existing ETT **(C, D)**, and a new ETT tube passed over the insertion tube. Endoscopic view with the distal tip of the insertion tube in the trachea at the level of existing ETT cuff **(E)**.

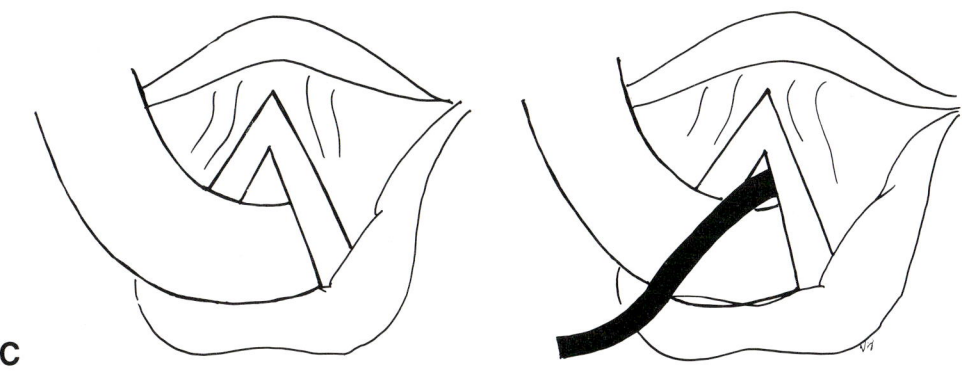

C

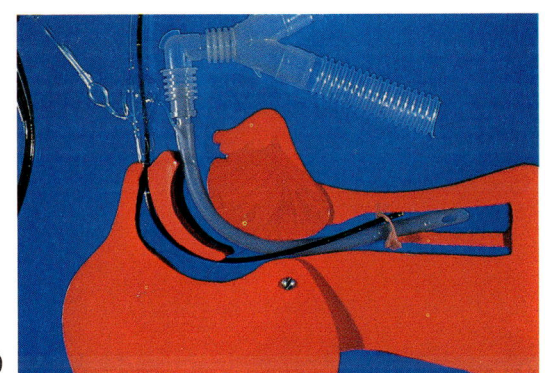

D

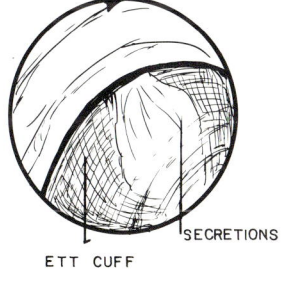

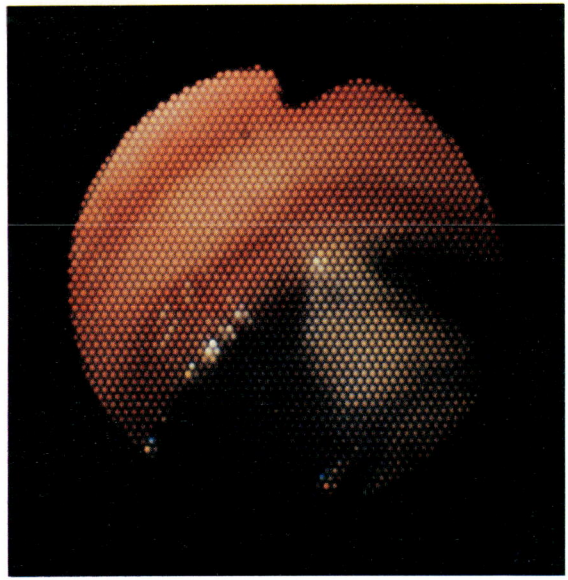

E

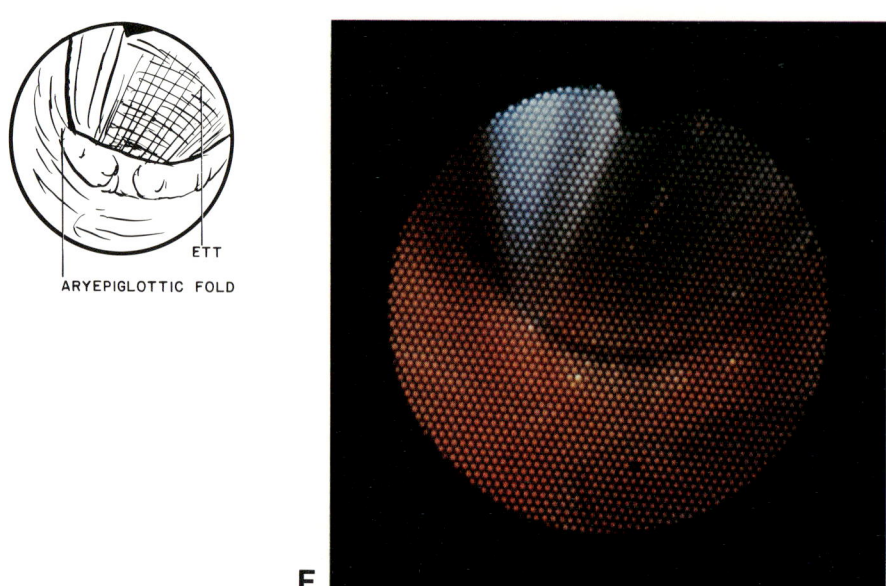

Fig 6–24. (cont.)—Endoscopic view of ETT fitting snugly in the posterior commissure **(F)**.

PERFORMING TRACHEOBRONCHIAL TOILET

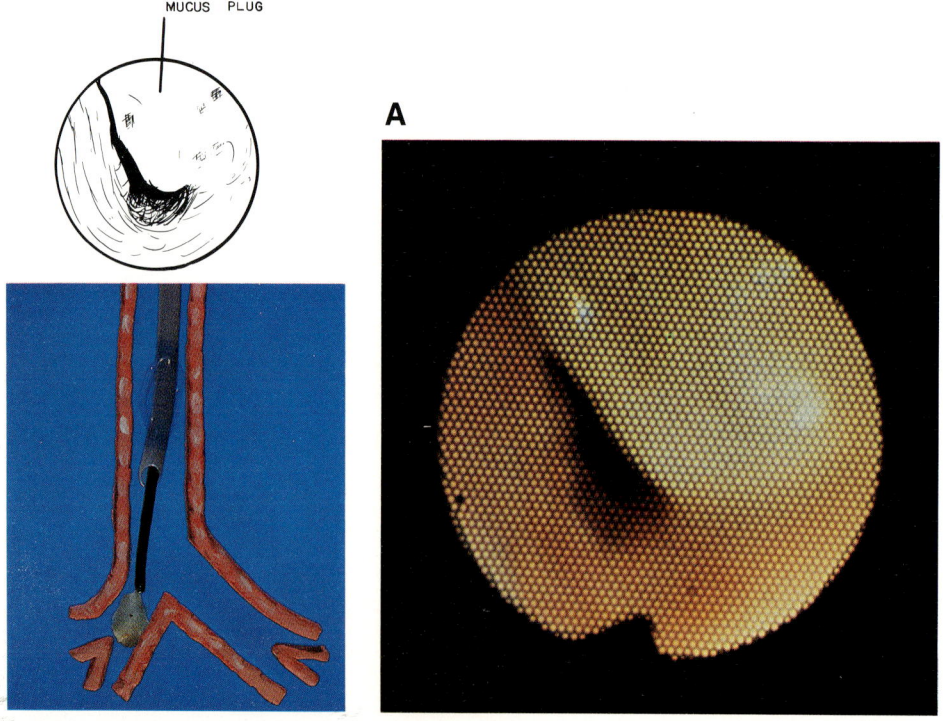

Fig 6–25.—The operating or suction channel may be used to remove mucus **(A)**, secretions **(B)**, and blood **(C)**. Suctioning may be performed in the operating room or intensive care unit.

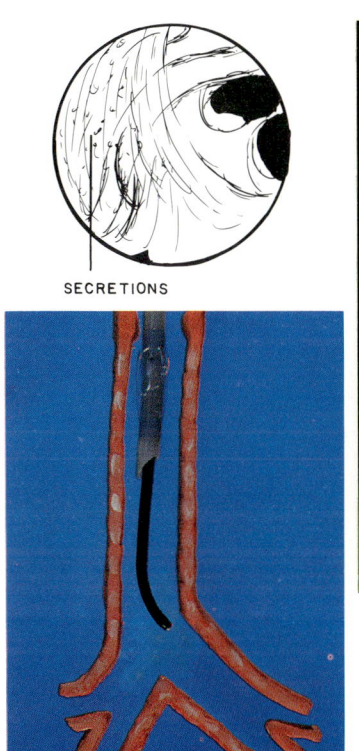
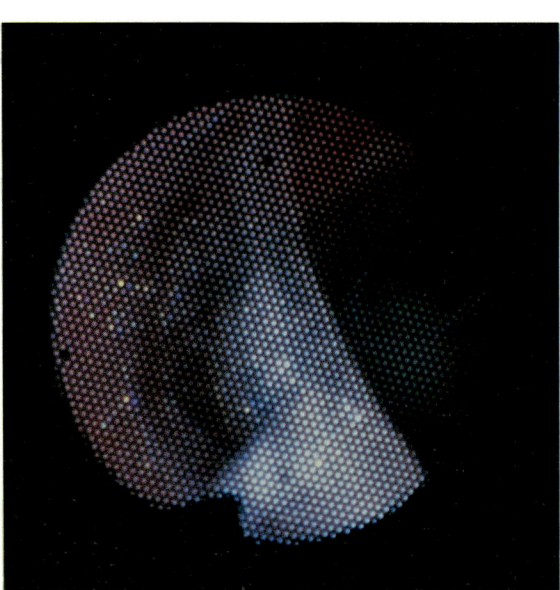

Fig 6–25 B.

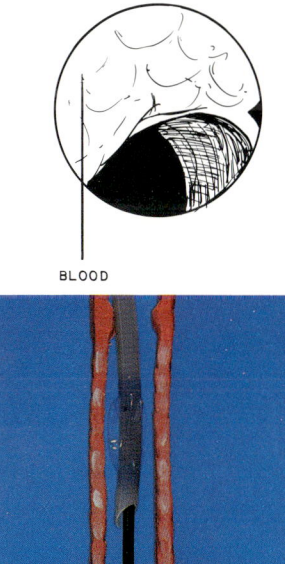
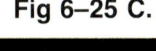

Fig 6–25 C.

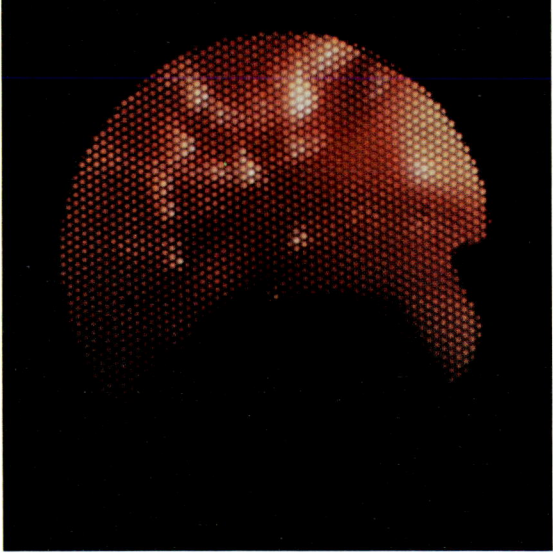

PLACING NASOGASTRIC TUBES

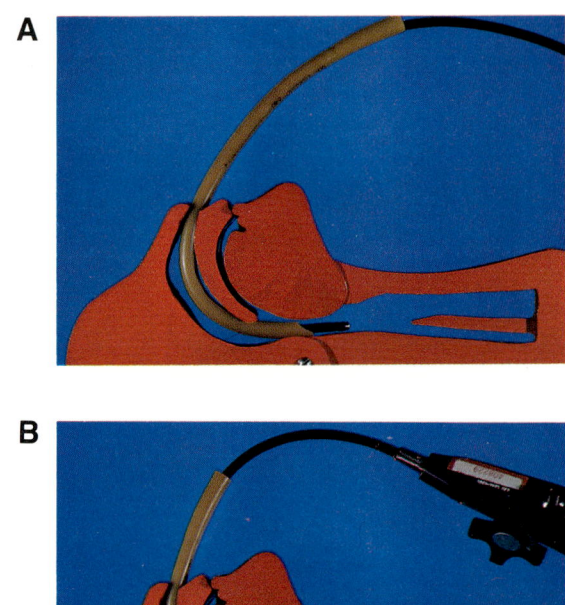

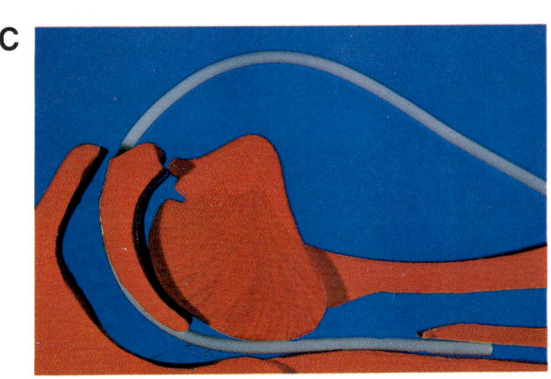

Fig 6–26.—Passage of nasogastric (NG) tubes may be difficult in obese, comatose, or anesthetized patients. The insertion tube of the endoscope is threaded into a longitudinally slit catheter **(A)** and advanced into the esophagus under direct vision **(B)**. The insertion tube is removed **(C)**, the NG tube threaded **(D)**, and the catheter removed. Endoscopic view of the esophagus **(E)**.

Fig 6–26 D.

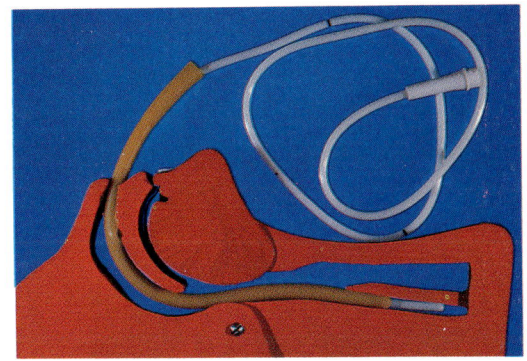

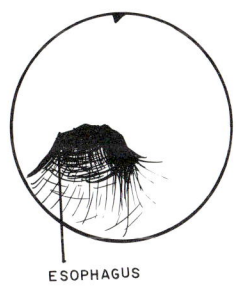

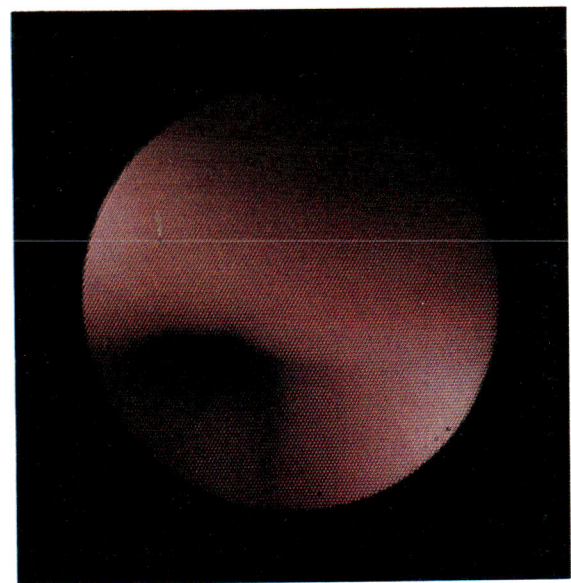

Fig 6–26 E.

Index

A

Adapter
  endoscopic, with port, 35
  oral airway with, 12, 30
Airway
  binasal, 12, 30, 105
  endoscopic, 87, 105, 107
  metal, 33
  nasal, 12, 31
  oral, 11–12
    with adapter, 12, 30
    Patil-Syracuse, 11–12, 29, 103
  pathology, evaluation of, 116–125
American Optical
  fiberoptic laryngoscope, 15
  fiberoptic stylet, 15
Anatomy, 43–73
  infant, 69–73
Anesthesia
  general, 37–39, 77, 78, 103–105
  local, 39–40, 106–110
  topical, 77
    atomizer for, 12, 34, 107
Angle
  bend
    mechanism, 24
    tip, 23
  bending, 84
Antifog agent, 9
Antisialagogues, 37
A-O Scientific Instruments fiberoptic adult bronchoscope, 19
Arrhythmias: cardiac, 39
Arthritis: juvenile rheumatoid, 124
Aryepiglottic folds, 49, 58, 89
  infant, 71
  inflammatory reaction of, 119
Arytenoids, 56
Atomizers, 12, 34, 107
Atropine, 37

B

Bending angle, 84
Binasal airway, 12, 30, 105
Bite block, 12, 33
Block (see Nerve, block)
Blood: in piriform fossa, 98
Bone, hyoid, position of, 48
  in child, 47
Bronchial blocker, 131
Bronchitis: chronic, 119
Bronchoscope, fiberoptic
  A-O Scientific Instruments, adult, 19
  Olympus
    adult, 18
    pediatric, 17
Bronchus
  lower lobe, 68
  main
    left, 65, 68, 129, 130
    left, segments of, 68
    right, 65, 66, 67
  superior lobe, 129
    right, 67
  upper lobe, 68

C

Camera
  with adapter, 20
  attachment, Olympus fiberoptic rhinolaryngoscope with, 16
  video, 21
Cardiac arrhythmias, 39
Care of instrument, 9–10, 21–25
  in test, 25
Carina, 65, 66, 96, 127
Cartilage
  corniculate, 49, 53, 56, 57, 58, 91
    infant, 71
  cuneiform, 49, 56
  thyroid, 64
  tracheal, 64, 65
Catheter: Fogarty, 131
Cervical spine, 125
Choledochoscope, 1
Cladding glass, 4
Cleaning, 10–11, 26
Clinical applications, 115–141

Cocaine, 37
Coherent bundle, 5
Commissure
　anterior, 62
　posterior, 61
Complications, 80–81
Connector: right-angle, 12, 30
Contractures: scar, 125
Core glass, 4
Corniculate cartilage, 49, 53, 56, 57, 58, 91
　infant, 71
Cricothyrotomy needle, 13, 35
Cuneiform cartilage, 49, 56
Cystic
　hygroma, 116
　lesions of vocal folds, 118

D

Defogging agent, 13, 34, 83
Diazepam, 40
Disinfection, 11
Distal lens, 5, 6
Double-lumen tube, 129–130
Droperidol, 40
Drugs: adjuvant, pharmacology of, 37–41

E

Edema, 121
Endobronchial tubes, 129–130
Endoscope: gas-sterilized fiberoptic, 21
Endoscopic
　adapter, with port, 35
　airway, 87, 105, 107
　mask, 11
　　Patil-Syracuse (*see* Patil-Syracuse mask)
Endotracheal tubes: changing, 135–138
Enflurane, 39
Epiglottis, 49, 52, 53, 54, 93, 97
　infant, 70
　position of, 48
　　in child, 47
Equipment
　ancillary, 11–13, 27–35
　preparation of, 83–87
Esophagus, 69

F

Facial nerve, 44
Failure: reasons for, 76–77, 97–100

Fentanyl citrate, 40
Fiber
　bundles
　　image-transmitting, 5
　　light-transmitting, 5
　damage, 22
Fiberoptic
　bronchoscope (*see* Bronchoscope)
　endoscope, gas-sterilized, 21
　laryngoscope (*see* Laryngoscope)
　laryngoscopy, guidelines for, 81
　rhinolaryngoscope, Olympus, with camera attachment, 16
　stylet, American Optical, 15
Fiberoscopes: Olympus Ultrathin, 19
Fibrous band, 122
Focusing, 84
Fogarty catheter, 131
Forceps: laryngeal, 12, 34
Fossa, piriform, 58, 59, 60
　blood in, 98

G

Gas
　sterilization, 11
　-sterilized fiberoptic endoscope, 21
Gauge: intubation, use of, 110–112
Glass
　cladding, 4
　core, 4
Glossopharyngeal nerve, 45
Glottis, 49, 57, 63, 92, 96
　infant, 70
Glycopyrrolate, 37
Goldenhar's syndrome, 116

H

Halo traction, 125
Halothane, 39
Hemorrhage, 121
Historical development, 1–7
Hygroma: cystic, 116
Hyoid bone, position of, 48
　in child, 47
Hypopharynx, 46
　anesthetized with atomizer, 107
　position of, 48
　　in child, 47

I

Image-transmitting bundle, 5
Incoherent bundle, 5
Infant anatomy, 69–73
Inflammatory reaction: of aryepiglottic
 and vestibular folds, 119
Inhalation injury, 118
Innovar, 40
Instrument care, 9–10, 21–25
 in test, 25
Instrumentation: available, 9, 13–21
Intravenous sedation, 40–41, 77
Intubation
 gauge, use of, 110–112
 nasotracheal, 78, 105–106, 109
  Patil-Syracuse mask for, 28
 orotracheal, 78, 104
  Patil-Syracuse mask for, 28
 prolonged, 122, 123
Isoflurane, 39

J

Juvenile rheumatoid arthritis, 124

L

Laryngeal
 atomizer, 12, 34
 forceps, 12, 34
 nerve (see Nerve, laryngeal)
 sinus, 63
 spray, McIntosh, 12, 34
Laryngoscope, fiberoptic
 American Optical, 15
 Machida, 16
Laryngoscopy
 fiberoptic, guidelines for, 81
 indirect, 38, 39
Larynx, 46, 88
Lens
 distal, 5, 6
 proximal, 6
Light
 source, 20
 -transmitting bundle, 5
Lubricant, 85

M

Machida fiberoptic laryngoscope, 16
McIntosh laryngeal spray, 12, 34

Mandible: receding, 124
Mannequin, 82
Mask, endoscopic, 11
 Patil-Syracuse (see Patil-Syracuse mask)
Maxillary branch: of trigeminal nerve, 44
Metal airway, 33

N

Narcotics, 40
Nasal airway, 12, 31
Nasogastric tubes, 140–141
Nasopharynx, 46
Nasotracheal intubation, 78, 105–106, 109
 Patil-Syracuse mask for, 28
Needle: cricothyrotomy, 13, 35
Nerve
 block
  laryngeal, internal, 77, 101
  techniques, 101–102
  transtracheal, 102
 facial, 44
 glossopharyngeal, 45
 laryngeal
  internal, block, 77, 101
  recurrent, 45
  recurrent, damage to, 120
  superior, 45
 trigeminal, maxillary branch of, 44
 vagus, 45
Nitrous oxide, 39

O

Olympus
 bronchoscope, fiberoptic
  adult, 18
  pediatric, 17
 rhinolaryngoscope, fiberoptic, with
  camera attachment, 16
 Ultrathin fiberoscopes, 19
Optical
 principles, 1–7
 stylet, Stortz, 14
Oral airway (see Airway, oral)
Oropharynx, 46, 55
 anesthetized with atomizer, 107
Orotracheal intubation, 78, 104
 Patil-Syracuse mask for, 28

P

Papillae, 50
Papillomatosis, 117
Patil-Syracuse
  airway, 11–12, 29, 103
  mask, 11, 27, 28, 103
    for nasotracheal intubation, 28
    for orotracheal intubation, 28
Pediatric fiberoptic bronchoscope: Olympus, 17
Pharmacology: of adjuvant drugs, 37–41
Pharynx, position of, 48
  in child, 47
Phenylephrine, 37
Physical characteristics, 2
Piriform fossa, 58, 59, 60
  blood in, 98
Plastic bite block, 33
Port: endoscopic adapter with, 35
Positioning, 79
Precautions, 80–81
Preparation: of equipment, 83–87
Prolonged intubation, 122, 123
Proximal lens, 6

R

Retractor: tongue, 12, 32
Rheumatoid arthritis: juvenile, 124
Rhinolaryngoscope: Olympus fiberoptic, with camera attachment, 16
Right-angle connector, 12, 30

S

Scar contractures, 125
Scopolamine, 37
Sedation: intravenous, 40–41, 77
Sinus: laryngeal, 63
Slit nasal airway, 12, 31
Soap: defogging, 13, 34, 83
Spine: cervical, 125
Sterilization, 10–11, 26
  gas, 11
Stortz optical stylet, 14
Stylet
  American Optical fiberoptic, 15
  Stortz optical, 14
Subglottic area
  anesthetized with atomizer, 107
  infant, 72

T

Teaching attachment
  for Olympus adult fiberoptic bronchoscope, 18
  for Stortz optical stylet, 14
Techniques, 75–113
Teeth, 51
Thyroid
  cartilage, 64
  gland, 116
Tongue, 43, 50, 52
  holders, 32
  retractor, 12, 32
Trachea, 64
  position of, 48
  in child, 47
Tracheal
  cartilage, 64, 65
  compression, 117
Tracheobronchial toilet, 138–139
Tracheostomies, 132–134
Traction: Halo, 125
Tranquilizers, 40
Transtracheal block, 102
Trigeminal nerve: maxillary branch of, 44
Tubes
  double-lumen, 129–130
  endobronchial, 129–130
  endotracheal, changing, 135–138
  nasogastric, 140–141
  placement, confirmation of, 126–130
Tumors, 116
Turbinates, 55

U

Uvula, 51, 53
  infant, 73

V

Vagus nerve, 45
Vasoconstrictors, 37
Vestibular folds, 49, 62, 63
  inflammatory reaction of, 119
Video camera, 21
Vocal folds, 49, 57, 60, 61, 63, 94, 99
  cystic lesions of, 118
  infant, 70, 71
  position of, 48
    in child, 47